W9-AOM-191

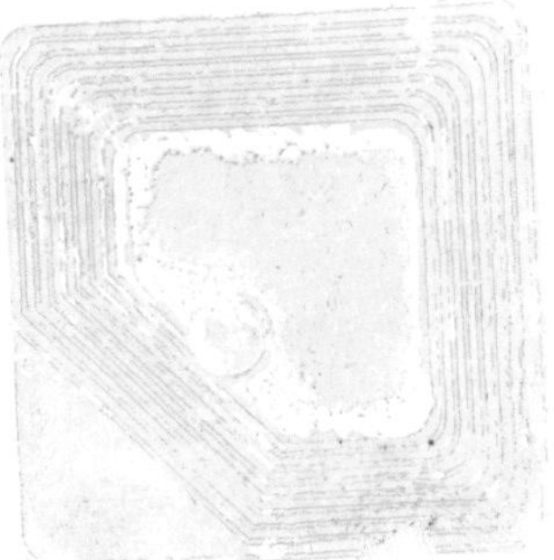

EAT RIGHT—ELECTROLYTE

EAT RIGHT—ELECTROLYTE

A NUTRITIONAL GUIDE TO MINERALS IN OUR DAILY DIET

W. REX HAWKINS, MD

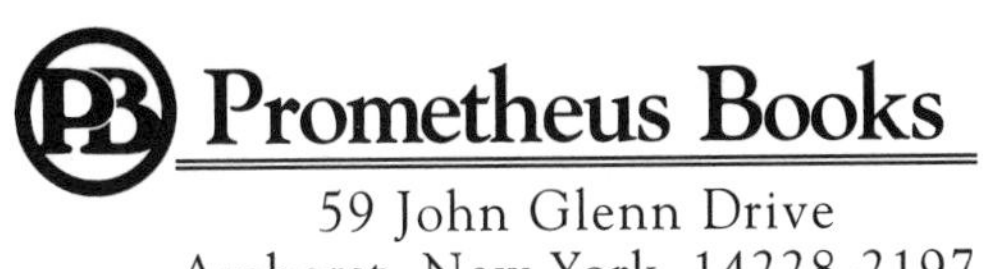

59 John Glenn Drive
Amherst, New York 14228-2197

Published 2006 by Prometheus Books

Inquiries should be addressed to
Prometheus Books
59 John Glenn Drive
Amherst, New York 14228–2197
VOICE: 716–691–0133, ext. 207
FAX: 716–564–2711
WWW.PROMETHEUSBOOKS.COM

10 09 08 07 06   5 4 3 2 1

Library of Congress Cataloging-in-Publication Data

Hawkins, W. Rex.
Eat right—electrolyte : a nutritional guide to minerals in our daily diet / W. Rex Hawkins.
p. cm.
Includes bibliographical references and index.
ISBN 1–59102–364–5 (hardcover : alk. paper)
1. Diet therapy. 2. Nutrition. I. Title.

RM217.H297189 2005
613.2'6—dc22

2005023839

Printed in the United States of America on acid-free paper

Dedication

At my grandmother's house at noontime, we had fried chicken, rice with gravy, a vegetable, biscuits or corn bread, and a dessert of freshly baked cookies or cake. I was very fond of fried chicken because my grandmother had been careful to pick one that was young and small. To fry chicken, to fix coffee, to boil rice, to make good biscuits and corn bread, and to cook vegetables with bacon and ham hock—that was my grandmother's specialty. I was always given my chosen piece of chicken, the leg usually. The others grabbed one or two pieces and my grandmother settled in with the gizzard and the back. She ate those bits because she loved us and did not want to take what we liked best—that was her charity.

Even at a young age I realized that my grandmother considered salt to be an essential ingredient in her cooking. No one complained, though. Tottie was acknowledged to be a master cook by all her friends and relatives. She was heavy, 165 pounds perhaps, but her good cheer and effusive spirit more than made up for any physical inadequacy imposed by the extra weight.

When she was seventy I realized that her facial expressions were less animated than they had been in the past and that her movements had slowed. And the next year, during our annual visit to her house, I noticed that her right arm and leg were partially paralyzed from a stroke she had experienced a few months earlier. In a conversation with my mom, my dad explained that my grandmother's physician had advised that she stop using salt. But, as he went on to say matter-of-factly, she had refused to do so.

My grandparents lived in a two-story house in rural central Florida. Grandmother commanded a spacious kitchen that contained many cabinets filled with foodstuffs of all kinds, pots, pans, dishes, and utensils of all sorts. Granddad, concerned about Tottie's decline in health and mindful of the physician's admonition, would hide the "When it rains, it pours" container in the far reaches of the kitchen. But my grandmother, despite her short stature, was always able to locate the "misplaced" salt container. At age seventy-five, almost five decades ago now, she died of high blood pressure and heart failure. Her health problems ignited a spark that led to my choice of medicine for a career. To her memory this book is dedicated.

CONTENTS

FOREWORD

Dr. Trevor C. Beard
Senior Research Fellow
Director, Salt Skip Program
Menzies Research Institute
Hobart, Tasmania 7000, Australia

Common salt (sodium chloride) is the world's oldest chemical food additive. The Industrial Revolution made it the cheapest, and today our supermarkets offer scarcely a single food without added salt, except for the fresh foods. This is curious, considering that this chemical food additive is completely unnecessary for perfect health.

No one adds salt to the diet of a breast-fed baby. Indeed it would be harmful—some salted foods tolerated by adults can even be fatal to young infants—yet few people realize that adults, too, can enjoy robust health from the cradle to the grave with an ideal diet of fresh fruit, vegetables, nuts, whole grains, and a little meat, poultry, and fish without adding a grain of salt.

As late as the middle of the last century about twenty "salt free" societies still existed, living in small tribal groups in isolated habitats on every continent except Antarctica. All without exception have detested salt when they first tasted it in foods that various explorers and anthropologists have shared with them. None have ever been offered salt as a public health measure, partly because there is no evidence that they need it, and partly because a Japanese research team recorded a rise in blood pressure in the Kalugaluvi people of Papua New Guinea within ten days of adding a "normal" amount of salt to their traditional diet.

An Australian medical expedition visited the Tukisenta people of Papua New Guinea in 1973, when their contact with the outside world was still very limited. Measured by the Harvard Pack Fitness Test, the salt-free locals of all ages were fitter than a team of fit young men from an Australian air force unit posted nearby.

The two elements that make up common salt—sodium and chloride—are called *electrolytes*. In the amounts found in breast milk and other natural (unsalted) foods, these two electrolytes are important nutrients, essential for life. Our grandmothers knew very well that perfect health requires a balanced diet, but something they overlooked when they cooked with salt was the overriding importance of the *electrolyte balance* in that balanced diet. Between 10 and 12 percent of the salt in the Western diet represents sodium and chloride as nutrients and the remaining 88 to 90 percent is salt being used as a chemical food additive. We eat about ten times more sodium and ten times more chloride than we need. Is that a balanced diet?

This highly readable book by Dr. Rex Hawkins is a timely reminder that electrolyte balance is no less important than the balance of all the other nutrients. For some conditions such as high blood pressure—treating it, checking its progress, or preventing it altogether—the electrolyte balance is crucial.

If you are concerned with health and longevity, Rex Hawkins has written a book you will find difficult to put down. This account of his voyage of discovery through the world of the dietary electrolytes will fascinate you, and you will profit greatly from it.

PREFACE

ELECTROLYTES

The chemical analysis of a food such as spinach shows that it is composed of water (85 percent) and the solid organic nutrients (15 percent): carbohydrates, fat, and protein. If we remove the latter compounds, we find a residual of minerals and vitamins. Water, carbohydrates, fat, protein, minerals, and vitamins are the essential nutrients.

A chemical analysis of one's body shows much the same thing. Assume a body weight of a hundred fifty pounds. Water weight would be about ninety pounds. Fat would be twenty-five pounds, more or less. The other thirty-five pounds would be protein (in muscle for instance), carbohydrates (the energy fuel within our body), and minerals (bones, teeth, and electrolytes).

This text stresses the importance of choosing foodstuffs that provide a proper balance of electrolytes. The latter can also be termed minerals. But there is a slight distinction. Minerals are inorganic materials found in the earth's crust. Electrolytes are compounds, including minerals, which when suspended in solution conduct a current of electricity.

Minerals are water-soluble. After birth, they enter our body in the form of electrolytes suspended and deposited in foodstuffs. Some electrolytes are positively charged—sodium, potassium, calcium, and magnesium, for example—whereas chlorine, phosphate, and sulfur ions are negatively charged.

Minerals are indestructible. They do not require special consideration during cooking. Once they enter the body they are there until excreted; they cannot be changed into anything else.

In general, electrolytes have two main functions. First, they can be an important constituent of the body in both the hard and soft tissues. For instance, clacium, magnesium, and phosphorous are very important in the structure of bones and teeth. And second, electrolytes are found in tissues and fluids of the body where they have functional roles.

Potassium is an integral part of muscles and various organs. Every cell of the body makes a continuous demand for electrolytes. Iron and phosphorous are found in every living cell—phosphorous in the nucleus and iron in the chromatin of the nucleus. Examples of electrolytes involved in the structure of the body are iodine in the thyroid gland, magnesium in the muscles and in blood cells, and copper in the liver and other tissues.

Electrolytes are also regulators of certain body functions. For example, sodium and potassium ions are important in the functioning of nerves. The transmission of a nerve impulse is facilitated by an exchange of sodium and potassium ions in the nerve cells. If the concentration of calcium, magnesium, sodium, and potassium in the fluids bathing nerve cells is altered, the ability to transmit nerve impulses will be disrupted.

The maintenance of the acid-base balance within the body is related to certain electrolytes. Some electrolytes have the capacity to generate an acid medium. They are predominant in protein foods like meats and eggs and in cereal products. Base-reacting electrolytes are found largely in fruits and vegetables. Diets that are rich in animal foods and low in vegetable foods, typical of industrialized countries, lead to a dietary net acid load that has a negative effect on calcium balance.

Another important function of electrolytes is their contribution to osmotic pressure and the movement of body liquids. The concentration of the major electrolytes within the body water—that is, sodium, potassium, and chlorine—governs the passage of fluids from one side of a membrane to the other. This process occurs when nutrients are carried by blood to various organs of the body. The fluids within and surrounding the cells of the body are regulated in a precise manner so that an osmotic equilibrium is maintained even while the body is undergoing a shift in electrolyte distribution.

The contractibility of muscles depends on the presence of calcium, sodium, potassium, and chloride in the fluid that bathes the muscle. This is especially true of that most important muscle, the heart. Calcium is essential to the rhythmic beating of that organ.

Electrolytes serve as catalysts in a number of important reactions that occur within the body. Examples are the catalytic action of enzymes in the metabolism of carbohydrates and fats and the clotting of blood by calcium.

The mineral elements required in macro amounts are calcium, chloride, magnesium, potassium, sodium, and sulfur. Those required in micro amounts are chromium, cobalt, copper, fluoride, iodine, iron, manganese, molybdenum, and selenium. In addition, there are several trace elements that appear to have biological functions. Elecrolytes seldom operate in isolation. They are interrelated and balanced to perform properly.

And that is the problem. The electrolytes ingested in our present-day diet are not balanced properly. That issue will be explored in the text material that follows.

AUTHOR'S ANALYSIS

The information presented herein is arranged in sequence to develop, step by step, the role that electrolytes/minerals play in the maintenance of good health. Included are sections detailing the obstacles that impede progress in achieving the recommended dietary guidelines. The text has been held to a minimum—the figures, the tables, the graphs, and the embedded data have been relied on to tell as much of the story as possible. It has been known for some time that high blood pressure, kidney stone, and osteoporosis, the three diseases placed center stage in the text, are a manifestation of an electrolytic imbalance within the body. But it had not been recognized until recent years that the role of dietary electrolytes in the development of those diseases, and for still others perhaps, is preeminent.

In 1997 and 2001, the DASH* Research Group released results in the *New England Journal of Medicine* which established that potassium, magnesium, and calcium have a lowering effect on blood pressure while sodium has the opposite effect. Earlier, in 1995, researchers at the University of Western Australia published data which showed that bone density changes in postmenopausal women correlated negatively with dietary sodium/salt intake while dietary calcium had the reverse effect. And in 2002, an Italian medical team published results which showed that kidney stone, a problem which was described in antiquity by Hippocrates, is due, at least in large part, to excessive dietary sodium and protein.

Those recent reports, and there are many others that support the same point of view, reflect a renewed interest by medical researchers in the field of dietary electrolytes. The public can be assured that still other diseases will come under the investigative

---

*Dietary Approaches to Stop Hypertension

microscope in time. In this book stomach cancer, Crohn's disease, and asthma are proposed as candidates for rigorous investigation.

Some might want medical research reporting to be focused elsewhere, while contending that diet is a personal matter undeserving of such attention. But that will not be the case. The researcher is an inquisitive individual. In the words of Louis Pasteur, the most notable chemist, scientist, and medical collaborator of the nineteenth century, the researcher will "exhaust every combination, until the mind can conceive no others possible."

For this book I, a retinal physician with undergraduate training in chemical engineering, have put ambiguity aside and attempted to talk up to the audience. The public thirsts for knowledge. I have tilled the landscape as seems appropriate for the moment. Not soon enough will someone furrow the field deeper and straighter. I eagerly await that time.

Acknowledgments

This book could not have been accomplished without the effort, enthusiasm, and selfless devotion of two people.

For many years now, A. Kathy Konkel, CRA, COT, has directed with great skill and tact the retina-vitreous practice for my associate, Dr. Burt Ginsburg, and myself. The results of Mrs. Konkel's and the staff photographer's efforts are apparent in the chapters that follow. In a second role, as the composition phase of *Eat Right—Electrolyte* was put in motion, Mrs. Konkel assumed the role of editorial assistant—the verification of source material, the compilation of references, and the production of the manuscript. Her assistance in all aspects of the finished product is gratefully acknowledged.

Mr. Michael A. Cooley, BS, AMI, a national award-winning illustrator, created the artwork, the effect of which more than satisfied the expectations of the author. The exactness of his execution lends greatly to the finished product.

Final kudos go to my wife, Edith, who is not only a distinguished pediatric pathologist but also an accomplished cook. Her expertise in the kitchen has made my self-imposed low-fat and 750 mg–sodium dietary regimen of the past thirty-two years a pleasant and enjoyable one.

CHAPTER 1

THE 1997 DASH* STUDY

LIFE EXPECTANCY DURING THE TWENTIETH CENTURY

In the twentieth century the life expectancy of Americans increased from forty-seven to seventy-seven, a thirty-year increment.[1] Much of that gain was the result of a substantial improvement in infant and childhood mortality made possible by the introduction of immunizations and antibiotics[2] and an equally impressive decrease in maternal mortality that followed the introduction of aseptic obstetrical care.[3] During that hundred-year interval, little was done, the statistics also reveal, to extend life beyond middle age. The improvement in life expectancy benefited children and young adults primarily, and women more than men.

The average middle-aged US adult of today does not live so

*Dietary Approaches to Stop Hypertension

very much longer than his or her counterpart did in 1900. Today's forty-five-year-old American male can look forward to living only five years longer, to age seventy-five, than his age mate did in 1900; and the forty-five-year-old American female of today lives only seven years longer, to age eighty, than her counterpart did at the turn of the twentieth century.[4] Those statistics reflect the fact that while older Americans of today have escaped fatal infections with immunizations, antibiotics, and sterilized operative techniques and with improved maternal mortality, they succumb prematurely and with great regularity to debilitating diseases which, oftentimes, suffer under the indictment of having been promoted by a lifetime of dietary indiscretions. Furthermore, those who survive to age seventy often spend the last years of their lives plagued by those same debilitating diseases, and by still other degenerative difficulties, all of which could have been minimized or prevented altogether by better lifestyle choices at an earlier age.

MAINTAINING GOOD HEALTH WITH DIETARY MEASURES

Physicians have long recognized that many medical problems can be ameliorated by dietary measures of one sort or another. Notable examples are the reduction of high blood pressure that follows a decrease in salt intake[5] and the amelioration of atherosclerotic cardiovascular disease that follows the elimination of dietary fats and cholesterol.[6] In the mid-1990s, dietary measures were subjected to still further scrutiny with an interventional dietary trial involving six medical institutions and sponsored by the National Heart, Lung, and Blood Institute of Bethesda, Maryland. Publication of the results followed in the May 7, 1997, issue of the *New England Journal of Medicine*.[7] The study, conducted by the DASH Research

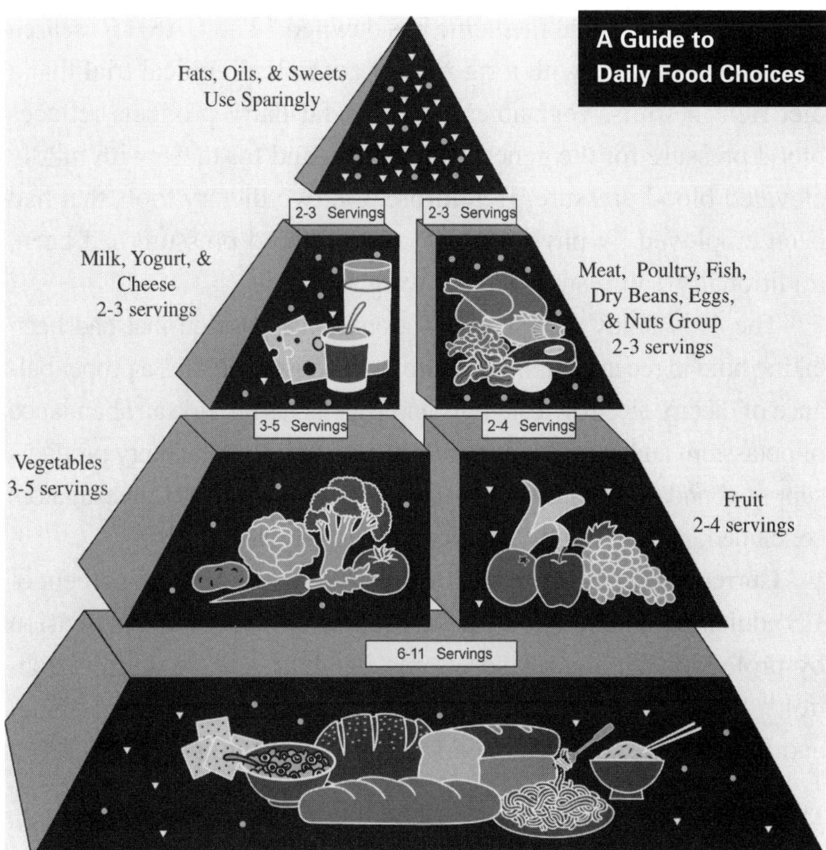

Fig. 1. United States Department of Agriculture Food Pyramid

Group, which comprised sixty-eight research physicians, nutritionists, and statisticians, documented the validity of a concept that had not been previously tested, and that is: When dietary sodium is maintained at a constant level, the types of food one eats and the electrolytic content of those foods can favorably influence an individual's blood pressure.

The 1997 study helped confirm the validity of an ideal food constituent pyramid,[8] anchored by fruits, vegetables, and grain products at the base (fig. 1). It is not an overstatement to say that a new era for nutritional medicine has dawned.[9] The DASH Research Group documented with a rigorously controlled clinical trial that a diet rich in fruits, vegetables, and low-fat dairy products reduces blood pressure for the general population and for those with mildly elevated blood pressure. Heretofore, the two dietary tools that had been employed by physicians to control blood pressure had been, traditionally, salt restriction and weight loss.

The 1997 study was an affirmation of the position that had been taking hold in recent years: blood pressure control requires a proper balance of dietary electrolytes. Fruits and vegetables provide an abundance of potassium and magnesium, and calcium, too. Low-fat dairy products supply abundant calcium. Those electrolytes, the DASH investigators concluded, play an important role in blood pressure control.

Currently it is estimated that fifty million people, or 25 percent of US adults, have high blood pressure (alternately termed hypertension by professionals) and of those, only one-half achieve optimal control.[10] It was in that context that the National Institute of Heart, Lung, and Blood released funds to perform the interventional trial.

METHOD OF STUDY FOR THE 1997 DASH TRIAL

The trial was designed to assess the effects of dietary patterns on blood pressure. Several hundred volunteer subjects with either normal or mildly elevated hypertension were recruited for a randomized feeding program at six US medical institutions. The food mix and fat-carbohydrate-protein profile for the test diets (tables 1 and 2) was as follows:

1. *Typical USA.* The typical US diet, which served as a control for comparative purposes, was representative of the foods consumed by a substantial number of Americans. The fat,

Table 1. Food Mix for Typical USA and Interventional Test Diets for the DASH Trial

Average Daily Servings, According to Diet

	*Typical USA**	*Enhanced Fruit/Vegetable*	*Enhanced Fruit/Vegetable Low-Fat*
Fruits and Juices	1.6	5.2	5.2
Vegetables	2.0	3.3	4.4
Grains	8.2	6.9	7.5
Low-fat Dairy	0.1	0.0	2.0
Regular-fat Dairy	0.4	0.3	0.7
Nuts, Seeds, and Legumes	0.0	0.6	0.7
Beef, Pork, and Ham	1.5	1.8	0.5
Poultry	0.8	0.4	0.6
Fish	0.2	0.3	0.5
Fat, Oils, and Salad Dressing	5.8	5.3	2.5
Snacks and Sweets	4.1	1.4	0.7

* Control diet, for comparison purposes

(Reproduced with permission from Appel, LJ et al. *New England Journal of Medicine* 1997;**336**:1117–1124)

Table 2. Fat-Carbohydrate-Protein Profile for Typical USA and Interventional Test Diets

	*Typical USA**	*Enhanced Fruit/Vegetable†*	*Enhanced Fruit/Vegetable Low-Fat‡*
Fat	36	36	26
Carbohydrate	50	49	56
Protein	14	15	18

*Control diet

†Fruits and vegetables enhanced; snacks and sweets reduced by 75 percent; total fat at 36 percent, identical to typical USA

‡Fruit, vegetable, and low-fat dairy products (milk, yogurt, etc.) enhanced; saturated fat products (cheese, processed meats, etc.) reduced; total fat at 26 percent

carbohydrate, and protein content, in calories, was 36, 50, and 14 percent, respectively.

2. *Enhanced Fruit/Vegetable.* This diet contained additional servings of fruits and vegetables and the elimination of most snacks and sweets. The fat, carbohydrate, and protein profile was intentionally maintained unchanged from that of the *typical USA* diet.
3. *Enhanced Fruit/Vegetable and Low-Fat.* This diet was rich in fruit, vegetables, and low-fat dairy products and had reduced amounts of saturated and total fat, including cholesterol. The fat, carbohydrate, and protein content, in calories, was 26, 56, and 18 percent, respectively.

Electrolytes

The electrolytic composition for the three diets is shown in table 3. Fruits and vegetables have an abundant amount not only of potassium and magnesium but also of calcium, as the analysis of the enhanced

Table 3. Electrolyte Content for Daily Servings of Interventional Test Diets*

	Typical USA	*Enhanced Fruit/Vegetable*	*Enhanced Fruit/Vegetable Low-Fat*
Sodium	3000	2900	2800
Potassium	2600	4100	4400
Magnesium	250	500	520
Calcium	300	400	1100

*Values are the results of chemical analyses of the menus prepared during the validation phase and during the trial. The sodium content for the enhanced fruit/vegetable diet, at 2900 mg, and the enhanced fruit/vegetable and low-fat diet, at 2800 mg, was less than the 3000 goal. That difference was of no significance as far as the final

diet indicates. The modified diet was additionally rich in calcium as a result of increased amounts of milk and low-fat dietary products.

Restrictions

During the course of the interventional trial, the researchers neutralized three lifestyle dietary variables that could affect the outcome. *Salt*, which has been shown in numerous studies to cause an elevation in blood pressure, was maintained at a 3000 mg level for each of the dietary regimens. *Weight*, which is positively (directly) associated with blood pressure and hypertension, was maintained at a constant level by daily caloric adjustment. And *alcohol*, which in both short- and long-term trials causes blood pressure to increase, was restricted to only one drink per week (table 4).

Table 4. Confounding Variables for DASH Intervention Trial

Sodium	daily adjustment to 3000 mg (approximately) per day
Weight	kept unchanged for each subject; controlled by caloric intake
Alcohol	restricted to one drink per week

Performance of Trial

The trial, managed by a professional team at each of the university testing centers, was conducted with a run-in and an intervention stage. The run-in phase was a three-week period during which all subjects were given the control (*typical USA*) diet. The volunteers, none of whom were taking medications, were then randomly assigned to one of the three diets and an eight-week intervention phase was begun. Blood pressure measurements were taken throughout the study period.

Results

The blood pressure for the control group remained unchanged throughout the entire study period. The *enhanced fruit/vegetable diet* participants, on the other hand, experienced a 2.8 mm Hg decrease in blood pressure. The *enhanced fruit/vegetable and low-fat diet* participants experienced a 5.5 mm Hg decrease (table 5)!

Table 5. Blood Pressure Change Following Eight Weeks Adherence to Interventional Test Diets

Diet	*Blood Pressure*
Control (Typical USA)	0
Enhanced Fruit/Vegetable	–2.2 mm Hg
Enhanced Fruit/Vegetable Low-Fat	–5.5 mm Hg

Observations

The study showed that dietary modification independent of sodium manipulation and weight loss can favorably affect blood pressure in adults. The reduction began soon after the interventional diets were commenced and was maintained throughout the duration of the trial. The investigators emphasized, in their discussion of the results, that the dietary modifications were not slight. An *enhanced fruit/vegetable diet* calls for 8 to 10 servings of fruits and vegetables per day as opposed to the 4.3 servings normally consumed by US adults (table 1). And the 2 to 3 servings of low-fat dairy products in the third diet are almost twice the average consumption of 1.5 servings per day.

In comparison to the *typical USA* diet, the potassium and magnesium levels for the interventional diets were increased by 70 to

100 percent. Calcium content was increased by 250 percent for the *enhanced fruit/vegetable and low-fat* diet (table 3).

Weight

During each phase of the dietary interventional trials, the DASH investigators maintained the weight of the subject volunteers at a constant level. A precaution of such type was necessary since there is overwhelming evidence of a positive relationship between blood pressure and body weight in adults. As early as 1969, a review article noted that more than thirty clinical studies published between 1929 and 1967 had confirmed the association. Since then, there have been additional reports in North America,[11] Australia,[12] Japan,[13] Sweden,[14] Britain,[15] and Holland.[16] A random population sample in two Belgian towns studied cross-sectionally (that is, with each age group equally represented) showed that a 2.2-pound rise in body weight was associated with a 2 mm Hg increase in blood pressure in men and a 3 mm Hg increase in women.[17]

Alcohol

The 1997 DASH study was distinguished further by the alcohol limitation that was imposed on the volunteers. Several studies have demonstrated an association between alcohol consumption and blood pressure in samples from the general population.[18] In most of the studies that have been reported, the blood pressure increase was greater at moderate levels (3–4 drinks per day) of alcohol consumption than at minimal levels (1–2 drinks per day). The increased effect on systolic blood pressure, for the moderate level of alcohol consumption, is 2–3 mm Hg or more.[19]

FALLOUT FROM THE DASH STUDY

The DASH Diet versus the Atkins-type Diet

Looking back, 1997 will be perceived as the turning point for the high-fat, high-protein, and low-carbohydrate Atkins diet and its clones. The DASH investigators swept Dr. Robert C. Atkins's concepts[20] aside and substituted a food mix anchored by fruits, vegetables, grain products, and low-fat dairy products (table 6). The US Department of Agriculture took heed of the 1997 study to bring its food pyramid into compliance (fig. 1).

At this juncture one might ask: How did the concept of the Atkins high-fat diet ever get started? Does not a high intake of dietary fat increase the cholesterol level within the blood? In a word—yes.[21] But human nature is such that a despondent and desperate individual suffering from a weight problem can be susceptible/vulnerable to cockamamie dietary schemes of whatever type.

It's not hard to devise an explanation to fit a set of circumstances. And that's what Dr. Atkins[22] did. He maintained that carbohydrates cause an increase in insulin production within the body. There's no argument there. That's the way the metabolism chain within the body is supposed to respond. But then he went on to say that insulin produced within the body promotes the storage of fat and leads to weight gain. At that point he stumbled. There are no scientific studies to substantiate such a claim.

During his thirty-plus years of practice, Atkins had ample opportunity and a sufficient number of clients to subject his diet to a clinical trial. But none was ever forthcoming.[23] He criticized with no small effect the American Medical Association for issuing an indictment of his *Diet Revolution* but did not offer statistics to counter its skepticism.[24]

Table 6. DASH Diet

Serving amounts are based on a diet of 2,000 calories per day

Food/Servings	*Servings Equals*	*Food Examples*
Grain products 7 daily	one slice of bread ½ cup dry cereal ½ cup cooked rice or pasta	whole wheat bread English muffin, pita bread, oatmeal, or grits
Fruits/vegetables	6 oz. fruit juice	apricots, bananas, grapes
5 fruit servings	one medium fruit	oranges, strawberries
4 vegetable servings	one cup raw or ½ cup cooked vegetables	peas, tomatoes potatoes, squash, leafy greens
Dairy foods (low-fat) 2 daily	8 oz. skim milk 1 cup yogurt 1½ oz. fat-free or lite cheese	skim or 1% milk low-fat yogurt part-skim cheese
Meats, poultry, and fish 1 to 2 daily	3 oz. cooked meat	lean meats only, trim visible fat broil, roast, or boil
Nuts, seeds, and legumes 1 daily	1/3 cup nuts ½ cup cooked legumes	almonds, peanuts kidney beans, lentils

Consider how the Atkins diet can be subjected to scientific evaluation: (1) Take, at baseline, the blood pressure and measure the serum cholesterol of a hundred or so volunteers (consecutive clients) at the Atkins Center for Contemporary Medicine in New York City. (2) Have one group follow the Atkins high-fat low-carbohydrate diet for eight weeks, while another group adheres to the average American diet, and, for good measure, have a third group adhere to a low-fat high-carbohydrate diet. *Adjust calorie content each day or two so that the weight of each subject volunteer remains unchanged. Maintain the same sodium dietary intake for each volunteer. Restrict alcohol.* Then, at the end of the eight-week period, measure each subject's blood pressure and serum cholesterol. For which diet can the blood pressure be expected to be lowest? The 1997 DASH trial showed that the low-fat diet will provide the lowest blood pressure. And other studies have shown that the cholesterol count will be the lowest for that diet.

What about the weight loss, or gain, with the Atkins diet? Weight is a function of caloric intake and exercise. Many diets work for a while because they call for the elimination of some food or other. The Atkins diet will promote weight loss if calories are reduced. What Dr. Atkins failed to acknowledge in each of his books, many of which were best-sellers, and during his public appearances, is that a dietary concept should promote good health first and foremost, and then, if desired, a pathway (caloric restriction) by which weight loss can be achieved.

The complete absence of scientific substantiation for Dr. Atkins's dietary concepts has been nothing more than appalling. He commanded a large following of patients after his ideas first attracted national attention in 1972. At this point one is surely entitled to ask: How much more time is needed before the high-fat low-carbohydrate concept of Dr. Atkins is subjected to scientific investigation?[25] And if no meaningful data are forthcoming from the Atkins Center for Contemporary Medicine or from other professional proponents, what is the justification for the high-fat, low-carbohydrate concept?

For many reasons the Atkins diet has been a big step backward. The absence of fruits, vegetables, and whole grains means less vitamins, oxidants, potassium, magnesium, calcium, and fiber. Many complain that the Atkins diet causes constipation and halitosis.[26]

Such symptoms can surely be annoying. But the more important concern is that excessive saturated fat and cholesterol provided by the diet surely clogs arteries, and that the electrolytes (potassium, magnesium, and calcium) excluded by a low-vegetable diet causes an increase in blood pressure.

Suzanne Somers and Other High-Fat High-Protein Proponenets

With her *New York Times* number one best-sellers *Eat Great, Lose Weight*; *Get Skinny on Fabulous Foods*; and *Eat, Cheat, and Melt the Fat Away*, Suzanne Somers, a television actress, has spread the word, with her coauthor, Dr. Dianna Schwarzbein, an endocrinologist, that losing weight and getting fit are easier now than ever before. Somers's concepts are similar to those of Dr. Robert Atkins, whom she applauds for having been the pioneer who took on the medical profession. Her criticism is directed pointedly at the food pyramid of the DASH Research Group. Following that dietary scheme, she says, "will only make [one's] body appear the same shape as a pyramid."[27]

Somers recommends that one should "turn the pyramid upside-down." When confronted with the question: "Isn't a low-fat diet the safest and most effective way to lose weight?" Her response was "Nooooooooooooooooooooooooooooo!" (By count, the reply was emphasized with seventy-five *o*'s). Somers explained that "we must eat protein and fat to make hormones that regulate the systems of the body and promote healthy cells." A low-fat diet, she insisted, is "dangerous to your health."

Really? The reverse proved to be the case, a short time later, as far as Somers's health is concerned. As *Eat, Cheat, and Melt the Fat Away* was being released, Somers divulged, on *Larry King Live*,[28] that she had developed a health problem of her own: breast cancer, which, fortunately, was successfully managed with surgery before the axillary lymph nodes had become involved.[29]

Somers's books have been best-sellers but they provide no scientific information. Dr. Carlon M. Colker,[30] author of *The Greenwich Diet: Lose Fat While Gaining New Health and Wellness*, goes down the same pathway of Atkins and Somers. He advocates not only an increased amount of fat in the diet but increased protein, too. To both his and Dr. Atkins's credit, cookies, cakes, pies, and similar products are shunned. Colker notes that "fat-free" cakes and cholesterol-free cookies have popped up on grocery shelves with increasing frequency during the past twenty-five years. Preying on the guilt of the public, cookie companies have attempted to create the impression that they produce a purified (cholesterol-free) product. With that sales approach, cakes and cookies have been flying off the grocery shelves as never before, to use Colker's phraseology, into the hands of gullible customers who sense that foods of such type meet, somehow, the minimal standard of medically acceptable nutrition.

Cookies, cakes, donuts, and the like provide little, if any, in the way of essential vitamins, fiber, and the necessary spectrum of electrolytes. Such foods were severely curtailed from the two interventional diets of the 1997 DASH study. It is instructive to point out that salad dressings, cakes, cookies, pie, candy, sweetened beverages, potato chips, and other calorie-dense, nutrient-sparse items were relegated to the upper portion (use only sparingly) of the food pyramid.

SUMMARY: LOW-FAT VERSUS HIGH-FAT

The Atkins, Somers, Colker, Tarnower (Scarsdale),[31] and Eades[32] diets, and others of similar type, substitute high-fat and "high-protein" foods for cookies, cakes, and other pastry products. The

DASH Research Group, on the other hand, substitutes fruits, vegetables, nuts, grains, and low-fat dairy products for such items. Both the DASH and the high-fat diet proponents share one commonality: they believe that cheap carbohydrates (cookies and the like) have no place in a healthy and nutritious dietary scheme.

NOTES

1. http://www.cdc.gov/nchs/data/lifetables/life89_1_3.pdf.

2. The death rate of smallpox in infants was 30 percent. See Zahorsky, J and Zahorsky, TS. *Synopsis of Pediatrics*. St. Louis: CV Mosby Co., 1953, p. 198. The mortality rate for diphtheria was 50 percent. See Vallery-Radot, R. *The Life of Louis Pasteur*. Garden City, NY: Doubleday, 1926, p. 456.

3. Kerr, JM and Johnstone, RW and Phillips, MH eds. *Historical Review of British Obstetrics and Gynaecology 1800–1950*. Edinburg and London: E & S Livingston Ltd, 1954. Chapter XXVI Puerpal Infections.

O'Doud, MJ and Phillip, EE eds. *The History of Obstetrics and Gynaecology*. New York: Parthenon Publishing Group, 1994. Chapter on Statistics—maternal mortality and perinatal mortality.

4. http://www.cdc.gov/nchs/data/lifetables/life89_1_3.pdf.

5. Morgan, T and Nowson, C. The role of sodium restriction in the management of hypertension. *Canadian Journal of Physiology and Pharmacology* 1986;**64**:786–796.

Australian National Health and Medical Research Council Dietary Salt Study Management Committee. Fall in blood pressure with modest reduction in dietary salt intake in mild hypertension. *The Lancet* 1989;**1**:399–402.

6. Ornish, D et al. Intensive lifestyle changes for reversal of coronary heart disease. *JAMA* 1998;**280**:2001–2007.

7. Appel, LJ and Moore, TJ and Obarzanek, E et al. A clinical trial of the effects of dietary patterns on blood pressure. *New England Journal of Medicine* 1997;**336**:1117–1124.

8. The food pyramid was originally conceived by the Agriculture Department in 1992 to reflect its recommendations. Following the 1997 DASH report the pyramid was modified to be in accordance with the latest available nutritional information. Additional adjustments can be expected from time to time. According to a August 30, 2004, report in the *Wall Street Journal*, the new recommendations from the Department of Agriculture are on the way: 7 servings of grains a day, instead of 9, and 10 servings of fruits and vegetables a day, up from 7.

9. In 1992 the US Department of Agriculture published revised (low-fat high-carbohydrate) dietary guidelines for Americans (USDA: *Nutrition and Your Health: Dietary Guidelines for Americans*. USDA Publication HG-232, 1992; *The Food Guide Pyramid*. USDA Publication HG-252, 1992) and included, for the first time, a food pyramid to illustrate the guidelines. Following the 1997 DASH study, the USDA pyramid was modified to conform more closely to that used by the DASH Research Group.

10. National High Blood Pressure Education Program Working Group report on primary prevention of hypertension. *Archives of Internal Medicine* 1993;**153**:186–208.

Stamler, J and Stamler, R and Neaton, JD. Blood pressure, systolic and diastolic, and cardiovascular risks: US population data. *Archives of Internal Medicine* 1993;**153**:598–615.

The sixth report of the Joint National Committee on Prevention, Detection, Evaluation, and Treatment of High Blood Pressure. *Archives of Internal Medicine* 1997;**157**:2413–2446.

11. Sims, EA. Mechanisms of hypertension in the overweight. *Hypertension* 1983;**4(Suppl III)**:III43–III49.

Dustan, HP. Obesity and hypertension. *Annals of Internal Medicine* 1985;**103(6 Pt 2)**:1047–1049.

12. Brennan, PS et al. The effects of body weight on serum cholesterol, serum triglycerides, serum urate and systolic blood pressure. *Australian and New Zealand Journal of Medicine* 1980;**10**:15–20.

13. Hiramatsu, K et al. Changes in endocrine activities relative to obesity in patients with essential hypertension. *Journal of the American Geriatrics Society* 1981;**29**:25–30.

14. Wilhelmsen, LW and Svärdsudd, KS and Berglund, GL. Development of high blood pressure and its consequence for health: a Swedish population study. In: *Epidemiology of Arterial Blood Pressure*. Kesteloot, H and Joossens, JV (eds.). The Hague: Martinus Nijhoff, 1980, pp. 311–324.

15. Bulpitt, CJ and Hodes, C and Everitt, MG. The relationship between blood pressure and biochemical risk factors in a general population. *British Journal of Preventative and Social Medicine* 1976;**30**: 158–162.

16. Florey, C duV and Uppal, S and Lowry, C. Relation between blood pressure, weight, plasma sugar and serum insulin levels in school children aged 9–12 years in Westland, Holland. *British Medical Journal* 1976;**1**:1368–1371.

17. Staessen, J et al. Four urinary cations and blood pressure: a population study in two Belgian towns. *American Journal of Epidemiology* 1983;**117**:676–687.

18. Kannel, WB and Sorlie, P. In: *Epidemiology and Control of Hypertension*. Paul, O (ed.). New York: Stratton Intercontinental Medical Book Corp., 1975, pp. 553–592.

19. Klantsky, WL et al. Alcohol consumption and blood pressure. *New England Journal of Medicine* 1977;**296**:1194–1200.

20. Atkins, RC. *Dr. Atkins' New Diet Revolution*. New York: Avon, 1997.

21. McGill, HC. The relationship of dietary cholesterol to serum cholesterol concentration and to atherosclerosis in man. *American Journal of Clinical Nutrition* 1979;**32**:2664–2702.

22. Dr. Robert C. Atkins died on April 17, 2003, following a fall. Earlier, in April 2002, he required hospital care for heart arrest. See Martin, D. Robert C Atkins, author of controversial but best-selling diet books, is dead at 72. *New York Times*. April 18, 2003, p. C13.

23. Medical literature search shows no published dietary studies for Dr. Robert C. Atkins.

24. Atkins, RC. *Dr. Atkins' Health Revolution*. New York: Houghton Mifflin Company, 1990, p. 5.

25. The fact that Dr. Atkins pursued the high-fat low-carbohydrate pathway without scientific validation was not lost to others. Note Dr. Dean Ornish's comment during a United States Department of Agriculture meeting in March 2000 (http://www.USDA.gov/cnpp), to wit, "Well, first of all, the last time I debated Dr. Atkins, I chided him for not publishing any research anywhere. . . ."

26. During the USDA debate (see above) mention was made that a group of people were placed on the Atkins diet in a controlled test situation. Later, Dr. Ornish noted that 65 percent of those participants reported halitosis and 70 percent were constipated. He goes on to explain, in his book *Eat More, Weigh Less* (foreword, p. xi): "When you eat a lot of meat, it takes a long time for it to make its way through your digestive tract. As it putrefies and decays, your breath smells bad, your sweat smells bad, and your bowels smell bad."

27. Somers, S. *Eat, Cheat and Melt the Fat Away*. New York: Crown, 2001.

28. http://www.cnn.com/TRANSCRIPTS/0103/28/1K1.00.html 81K.

29. One cannot but wonder if the hormone replacement therapy that Somers steadfastly adhered to for many years (and had recommended to her readers—"When estrogen levels are lowered you are more susceptible to weight gain") had made her vulnerable to the development of breast cancer. A second consideration is the high-fat diet itself. In recent decades the high fat content for the diet of Western world countries has been incriminated as a risk factor for breast cancer (see Mettlin, C. Diet and the epidemiology of human breast cancer. *Cancer* 1984;**53**:605–611). During the *Larry King Live* interview, Somers emphasized, interestingly, that she would not be deterred, because of the breast cancer, from continuing hormonal replacement therapy. And there would be no dietary changes, she also went on to say.

The breast cancer information was released, in March of 2001, at the time of an even more startling revelation: Somers had developed a weight problem and had opted for liposuction at the Lasky Clinic in Beverly Hills, California. According to the initial news source, the *National*

Enquirer, and the text of the *Larry King Live* interview, liposuction was done to her thighs, abdomen, hips, and upper back. Somers's dietary fans were surely perplexed by such news. The upside-down pyramid advocate had encountered a weight problem in addition to her episode with cancer.

30. Colker, CM. *The Greenwich Diet*. New York: Advanced Research Press, 2000.

31. Dr. Tarnower, the originator of the Scarsdale diet, died in 1980.

32. Eades, MR and Eades, MD. A new nutritional perspective. In: *Protein Power*. New York: Bantam Books, 1996, pp. 3–18.

CHAPTER 2

THE 2001 DASH STUDY

EFFECTS ON BLOOD PRESSURE OF REDUCED DIETARY SODIUM

The 1997 DASH study excluded lifestyle factors that have an effect on blood pressure: daily sodium (salt) intake, weight loss/gain, and alcohol consumption. During the eight-week interventional dietary period, caloric intake was adjusted daily. Alcohol consumption was prohibited. Daily sodium intake was maintained at 3000 mg.

Sodium Restriction Comes Under Attack

Following publication of the 1997 DASH study, some medical scientists interpreted the findings as indicating that salt restriction might not be very important for either the control or the treatment of high blood pressure. Nick Davy, a medical professional and head of the biostatistical unit of the British Medical Research Council, summarized that view to Gary Taubes, a technical writer.[1]

> The (1997) DASH results suggest that fruits and vegetables may be the cause of effects attributed to salt in the old ecologic studies. Societies that have high salt intake tend to consume highly salted preserved foods simply because they do not have access to fruits and vegetables.

For decades medical physicians had accepted, on the basis of abundant clinical and laboratory research, the proposition that dietary salt is hazardous to one's health and blood pressure. In the early 1990s, though, that thesis had come under attack. The clinical trials and animal experiments that had been used to indict salt were questioned.[2] High blood pressure came to be recognized as a complex problem with risk factors other than salt responsible for its development.[3]

Some became willing to greatly diminish, if not completely reject, the role of salt as a causative factor for high blood pressure/hypertension.[4]

Taubes interviewed more than eighty researchers, clinicians, and administrators following publication of the 1997 DASH trial. He concluded, in an extensive August 14, 1998, *Science* journal review,[5] that the available data up to that time did not support a forceful recommendation regarding dietary salt usage.

> After decades of intensive research, the apparent benefits of avoiding salt have only been diminished. This suggests that either the true benefit has now been revealed and it is indeed small, or that it is nonexistent, and researchers believing such benefits have been deluded by the confounding influences of other variables.

Drummond Rennie, a *JAMA* (*Journal of the American Medical Association*) editor and University of California, San Francisco physiologist, extended the criticism in that same issue of *Science*.

He felt that the National Heart, Lung, and Blood Institute had demonstrated, with its support of the 1997 DASH trial and similar studies during the past two decades, "a commitment to salt education that goes way beyond the scientific facts."

Jeremiah Stamler, a cardiologist at Northwestern University Medical School in Chicago, contended, on the other hand, that any controversy regarding salt has "no genuine scientific basis in reproducible fact." He felt that the indictment against salt was irrefutable. "The appearance of controversy among medical researchers," he said in *Science*, in 1998, "permits the food industry to mount an orchestrated resistance," which he likened to the "obfuscation created by the tobacco industry in the fight over cigarettes." He went on to say, "My considerable experience is that there is no scientific interest on the part of these people [the food industry] to tell the truth."

Mindful that sodium's role as a hypertensive risk factor required better definition, the National Heart, Lung, and Blood Institute administrators opted for additional dietary studies. In 1998 they authorized funds for a trial in which sodium would be the sole dietary variable. Any uncertainty that Davy, Taubes, Rennie, and others might have had about sodium's effect on blood pressure was soon to be resolved.

Methodology for 2001 DASH Study

Like its predecessor, 2001 DASH was a multicenter randomized controlled feeding trial. The goal was to compare the effect of three levels of dietary sodium on blood pressure in people eating either a typical USA diet or the DASH enhanced fruit/vegetable and low-fat diet. In contrast to the 1997 DASH trial, during which the sodium level was maintained at 3000 mg daily, the new trial provided for the sodium level to be reduced in steplike fashion from a high (3500 mg), to an intermediate (2300 mg), and, finally, to a low (1150 mg) level.

The 3500 mg initial level was thought to be representative of the average sodium intake for the US populace.[6]

Again, several hundred people were recruited for the trial. The study population had systolic blood pressure readings in the 120 to 159 mm Hg range; 57 percent of the volunteers were women; 57 percent were black. Average age was forty-eight. The group was generally healthy, with an absence of heart disease, kidney insufficiency, and diabetes.

The trial commenced with a two-week run-in period during which all participants ate a typical USA diet with a 3500 mg sodium content. Then, the participants were randomly assigned, for a thirty-day period, to either (1) a typical USA group or (2) a DASH (enhanced fruit/vegetable and low-fat) group, following which the dietary trial continued for additional thirty-day periods at, first, the 3500 mg sodium level, then the 2300 mg level, and, finally, the 1200 mg level.

Results (New England Journal of Medicine, January 2001)[7]

At each level of sodium intake—high, intermediate, and low—the blood pressure was lower for patients following the DASH diet than for those assigned to the control (typical USA) diet.

The trial confirmed, at onset, the efficacy of the DASH diet for maintaining a low blood pressure (table 1 and fig. 1). At the 3500 mg level, the blood pressure was 5.9 mm Hg less for the DASH group. At the 2300 mg level, the blood pressure decreased 2.1 mm for the typical USA group and 1.3 mm for the DASH group. Reduction of sodium intake to 1150 mg resulted in an additional lowering of 4.6 mm for the typical USA group and 1.7 mm Hg for those on the DASH diet. The effect of sodium was observed in participants with and in those without hypertension, in blacks and those of other races, and in women and men.

Comparison of the typical USA diet at the high (3500 mg)

Table 1. The Blood Pressure Effect of Reduced Sodium Intake

Diet Group	*3500 mg*	*2300 mg*	*1150 mg*	*Total Effect (mm Hg)*
Typical USA	—	–2.1	–4.6	–6.7
DASH	–5.9	–1.3	–1.7	–8.9

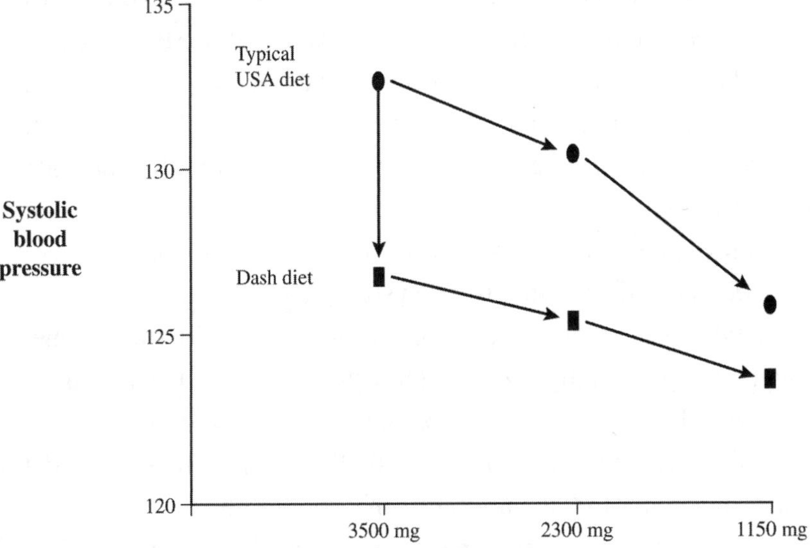

Fig. 1. The effect on systolic blood pressure of reduced sodium intake and DASH diet. When half of the subjects were switched from the typical USA diet to the DASH diet (vertical arrow), systolic blood pressure decreased by 5.9 mm Hg. Then, as dietary sodium was withdrawn for both groups, the blood pressure decreased for each group to a lower level. (Modified and reproduced by permission from the *New England Journal of Medicine* 2001;**344**:3–9, copyright 2001 Massachusetts Medical Society)

sodium level and the DASH diet at the low (1150 mg) sodium level showed a blood pressure reduction of 8.9 mm Hg for the DASH diet. That amount is similar, the authors emphasized, to the improvement achieved from blood pressure–lowering drugs. The blood pressure for the typical USA group decreased 6.7 mm Hg as the sodium content was reduced to 1150 mg.

OVERVIEW

For the proponents of dietary control of hypertension, 2001 DASH-sodium was another spectacular success. To start, the study confirmed the 1997 DASH findings. Systolic blood pressure fell 5.9 mm Hg as the diet was switched to enhanced fruit/vegetable and low fat.[8] In addition, the study confirmed the results of prior clinical trials of the past fifty years which had showed that dietary restriction of sodium is an effective means of reducing blood pressure.

2001 DASH-sodium provided strong evidence that both sodium reduction and an enhanced fruit/vegetable low-fat diet, alone or together, significantly reduce blood pressure. The US Department of Agriculture recommendation has been 2400 mg daily, until recently. According to the August 30, 2004, *Wall Street Journal*, the panel advising the departments of Agriculture and Health and Human Services has recommended a slightly lower limit of 2300 mg. After toying with a 1500 mg recommendation, the panel backed away from such stringent advice and allowed the salt-industry advocates and snack-food makers to breathe a sigh of relief. According to the *Wall Street Journal* account, the government was afraid a 1500 mg recommendation would cause a market upheaval similar to what the government's low-fat recommendations spurred years ago.

The 1997 DASH trial showed that the increase in dietary potassium, magnesium, and calcium—a result of the fruit and vegetable enhancement—causes a very substantial reduction in blood pressure. The 1997 DASH diet was also low in fat, which proved to be an additional assist for blood pressure. The 2001 DASH-sodium trial showed that low sodium intake causes an additional decrease in blood pressure. The combined effect was not as great as would be estimated on the basis of separate contribution, but was quite substantial, nevertheless.

The two studies showed that blood pressure is ameliorated by increased amounts of dietary potassium, magnesium, and calcium and decreased amounts of dietary sodium.

The Duke (Kempner) Rice Diet, the Pritikin, and the Ornish Programs

The 2001 DASH-sodium diet was not a new concept. Earlier, the American Heart Association[9] and the US Dietary Guideline Committee[10] had advocated a low-fat, high-carbohydrate, and low-sodium food pyramid of similar type. And, much earlier, in the 1940s, a low-fat and low-sodium regimen had been improvised at Duke University under the direction of Dr. Walter Kempner.[11] That scheme became known as the Rice Diet Program.[12]

In the 1960s, Nathan Pritikin, an engineer/inventor, began a longevity program similar to Duke's, in Santa Monica, California.[13] Today, the Pritikin program is located at Adventura, Florida.[14]

Finally, the Ornish program in Sausalito, California, which began operation in the 1980s, advocates a dietary plan similar to 2001 DASH-sodium.[15]

Supervised dietary and exercise programs are provided at those centers for patients/clients who may be experiencing a disabling health problem: heart failure, diabetes, hypertension, obesity, and the like. For the first couple of weeks a rigorous dietary program is maintained. Then, as clinical improvement becomes evident and the exercise program is lengthened, the caloric and sodium intake is increased.

The Duke Rice Diet Program is perhaps the most demanding. For the first couple of weeks calories are limited to 700 and sodium to 25 mg! For the second two-week period the calories are increased, typically, to 1100 and sodium to 250 mg.

The physicians with the Rice Diet Program recommend a more liberal diet to be followed on returning home. Likewise, for Pritikin and Ornish. The characteristics of the maintenance diet for each of these regimens approach those of the 2001 DASH-sodium diet.

The dietary and exercise program at those facilities and others like them produces remarkable results in a short period of time. The Rice Diet Program was started in 1944 under the direction of Walter Kempner, MD (1903–1997). He was an émigré from Germany (in 1934). Initially, in the 1940s and 1950s, the patients referred to the Duke program had terminal kidney and heart failure and/or malignant hypertension (systolic blood pressure of 220 or more). Few medications were available at that time for such problems. Diet was the only option.

Kempner was the first to show that blood cholesterol can be lowered by dietary modification. In 1953 he reported the results for eight hundred patients who when first seen had prominently elevated blood cholesterol (among other problems). Following a 120-day dietary program, the cholesterol decreased, on average, from 283 to 205![16] Subsequent studies at Duke have consistently demonstrated remarkable results for patients with hypertension, diabetes (especially those with retinopathy), kidney failure, obesity, and heart failure.[17]

In contradiction to the silent pen of Atkins, Colker, Eades, and others who have advocated a high-fat and high-protein diet, the Rice Diet, Pritikin, and Ornish camps have placed numerous scientific reports in peer-reviewed journals. In a series of extraordinary reports,[18] Ornish, in collaboration with L. Gould and others, showed that a low-fat, high-carbohydrate, and low-sodium diet, along with stress management and exercise, can reverse cholesterol plaques within coronary arteries and improve blood flow to the heart muscle of atherosclerotic subjects. Severe coronary artery obstruction (stenosis) has been relieved for individuals who vigorously modified dietary risk factors.

Recently, a groundbreaking report from the Pritikin program has established a link between prostate cancer and diet. A rigorous low-fat, high-carbohydrate diet was found to reverse prostate cancer for a high percentage of subjects so afflicted. "To my knowledge, this is the first study which documents that dietary changes and exercise might in fact kill prostate cancer cells," said lead investigator Dr. James Barnard of UCLA.[19] The Pritikin and Ornish programs are the subject of separate texts.[20]

VEGETARIANISM AND SODIUM

When animal products are excluded from the diet, the fat content is often decreased by a considerable degree. And protein is reduced, too. But salt content might not be at a low level, especially if one is not discriminating in the purchase of items such as cereals, soups, sauces, and salad dressings, for instance, and if cheese is included in the diet. A vegan diet does not necessarily comply with the specifications of the 2001 DASH-sodium concepts. The comparison would depend particularly on what provisions are made regarding sodium content.

NOTES

1. Taubes, G. The (political) science of salt. *Science* 1998; **281**:898–907.

2. Alderman, MH et al. Association of the rennin-sodium profile with the risk of myocardial infarction in patients with hypertension. *New England Journal of Medicine* 1991;**324**:1098–1104.

3. Tobian, L. Potassium and hypertension. *Nutrition Reviews* 1988;**8**:273–283.

Whelton, PK and Klag, MJ. Magnesium and blood pressure: review of the epidemiologic and clinical trial experience. *American Journal of Cardiology* 1989;**63**:26G–30G.

4. Kagan, A et al. Dietary and other risk factors for stroke in Hawaiian Japanese men. *Stroke* 1985;**16**:390–396.

Khaw, KT and Barrett-Connor, E. Dietary potassium and stroke-associated mortality: a 12-year prospective population study. *New England Journal of Medicine* 1987;**316**:235–240.

5. Taubes, G. The (political) science of salt. *Science* 1998;**281**: 898–907.

6. See INTERSALT study. *British Medical Journal* 1988;**297**:319–328.

7. Sacks, FM et al. for the DASH-Sodium Collaborative Group. Effects on blood pressure of reduced dietary sodium and the dietary approaches to stop hypertension (DASH) diet. *New England Journal of Medicine* 2001;**344**:3–10.

8. In the 1997 DASH study, systolic blood pressure decreased 5.5 mm Hg when subjects were switched from the typical USA to the DASH diet.

9. American Heart Association. The healthy American diet. *Circulation* 1991;**82**:1079.

10. US Dietary Committee, US Department of Agriculture, US Department of Health and Human Services. *Nutrition and Your Health: Dietary Guidelines for Americans.* 4th ed. 1995. *Home & Garden Bulletin* 232.

11. Kempner, W. Treatment of heart and kidney disease and of hypertensive and arteriosclerotic vascular disease with the rice diet. *Annals of Internal Medicine* 1949;**31**:821–856.

12. Rosati, KG. *Heal Your Heart.* New York: John Wiley, 1997. http://www.RiceDietProgram.com.

13. Pritikin, R. *The New Pritikin Program.* New York: Simon & Schuster, 1990.

14. http://www.Pritikin.com.

15. Ornish, D. *Eat More, Weigh Less*. New York: Quill, 2001. http://www.Ornish.com.

16. Kempner, W. Radical dietary treatment of hypertensive and arteriosclerotic vascular disease, heart, and kidney disease, and vascular retinopathy. *General Practitioner* 1954;**9**:71–93.

17. The scientific publications of Dr. Kempner between 1927 and 1941 have been compiled by Dr. Barbara Newborg, his longtime associate, and, in 2002, printed (reproduced) in text format by Gravity Press of Durham, North Carolina. The final paragraph of Dr. Newborg's foreword, which reviews Dr. Kempner's research activities in the 1930s, reads as follows: "Kempner's experiments with kidney tissues under conditions of low oxygen tension led to his epoch-making and far-reaching medical discovery: the use of a radical dietary treatment to compensate for renal metabolic dysfunction. The diet consists of about 95% carbohydrates, with the virtual elimination of sodium and fat, and a minimum of animal protein. It includes high potassium levels and low chloride. The so-called rice diet also brought about other dramatic and unanticipated results: decrease in heart size, compensation of heart and kidney failure, restoration of eyesight to blind patients, improvement in diabetic patients." The papers authored by Dr. Kempner subsequent to 1941 were published by Gravity Press in 2004.

18. Gould, KL et al. Improved stenosis geometry by quantitative coronary arteriography after vigorous risk factor modification. *American Journal of Cardiology* 1992;**69**:845–853.

Gould, KL et al. Changes in myocardial perfusion abnormalities by positron emission tomography after long-term, intense risk factor modification. *JAMA* 1995;**274**:894–901.

Ornish, D et al. Can intensive lifestyle changes reverse coronary heart disease? 5-year follow-up of the Lifestyle Heart Trial. *JAMA* 1998;**280**:2001–2007.

19. http://www.uclanews.ucla.edu.

20. Pritikin, R. *The New Pritikin Program*. New York: Simon & Schuster, 1990.

Ornish, D. *Eat More, Weigh Less*. New York: Quill, 2001.

CHAPTER 3

HIGH BLOOD PRESSURE, GENERAL CONSIDERATIONS

Just how important is the 8.9 mm Hg reduction in blood pressure that can be realized by switching from the typical USA to the DASH–1150 mg sodium diet? The answer to that question begins with a consideration of the heart.

HEART

The work performed by the heart is considerable. At an average rate of seventy-two contractions per minute, the heart pumps blood, a viscous fluid containing cells and particulate matter, through the arteries of the body and into the capillaries. The blood streams rapidly through the arteries, but the capillaries, which are small in size, dampen the flow to a considerable degree. The slowing allows nutrients and other substances to diffuse into the surrounding tissues and back again. Next, the flow moves passively into the veins, which serve as a return conduit to the heart.

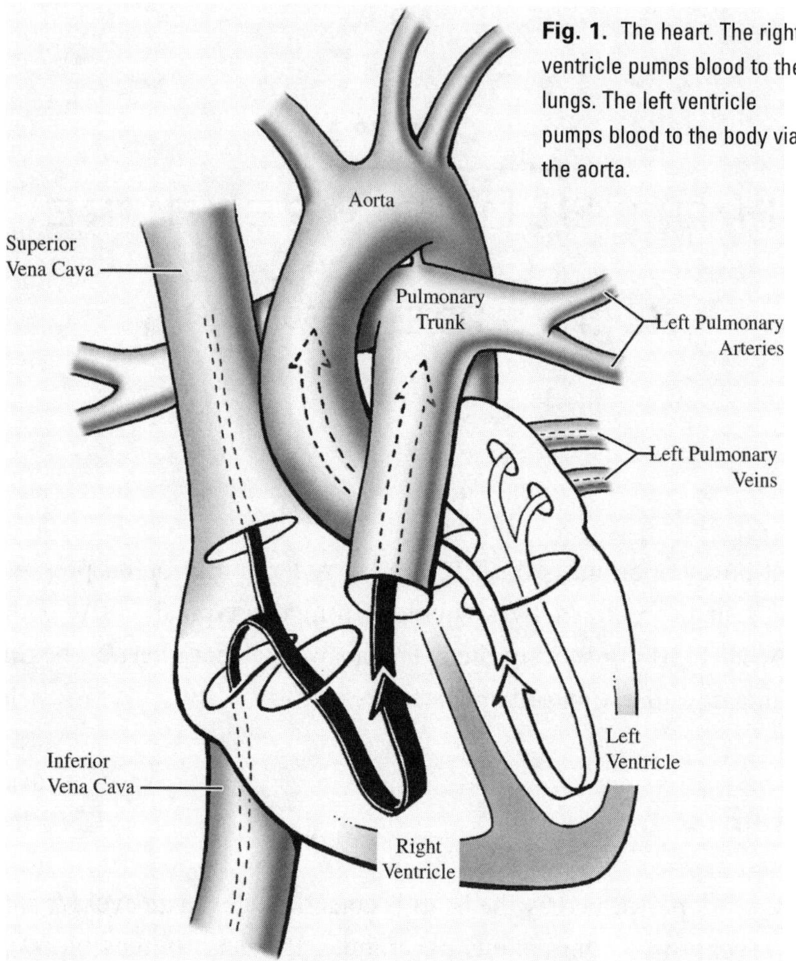

Fig. 1. The heart. The right ventricle pumps blood to the lungs. The left ventricle pumps blood to the body via the aorta.

The heart has two sides, a right and a left, the contractive chamber for which is called the *ventricle* (fig. 1). The right ventricle has the task of sending blood through the lungs where carbon dioxide is exchanged for oxygen. The left ventricle receives the oxygenated blood from the lungs and then commences another cycle by propelling blood into the *aorta*, the primary artery of the body.

Blood Pressure, Defined

As blood is propelled into the arterial system, the larger vessels expand slightly to accommodate the increased volume (fig. 2). At that moment the blood pressure is maximal, the so-called systolic pressure. Instantly, the valves between the left ventricle and the aorta close so that the blood flow proceeds forward into the smaller arteries and, ultimately, into the capillaries.

As the heart relaxes, filling of the chambers occurs. Blood from the veins flows into the right ventricle. Blood from the lungs fills the left ventricle. During that brief interval the blood pressure is at its lowest level, the so-called diastolic pressure.

Work of the Heart

It has been determined that the pumping of the heart muscle accounts for 20 percent of the work performed (the energy expended) by the body during an average day. Energy is also required for the contractions of the digestive tract, which allows for the passage of nutrients into the blood stream, for the respiratory (breathing) muscles, and for the metabolic activity of each cell within the body. Finally, energy is expended by the muscles that perform the physical activities of working, chewing, sitting, lifting, and running.

The work of the heart is influenced to a considerable degree by the blood pressure level. The higher the blood pressure, the greater is the work of the heart. It should be apparent that the 8.9 mm Hg reduction in blood pressure that can be produced by adherence to the 2001 DASH–1150 mg sodium diet would significantly decrease the contractile force required of the heart. Assume a 120/80 blood

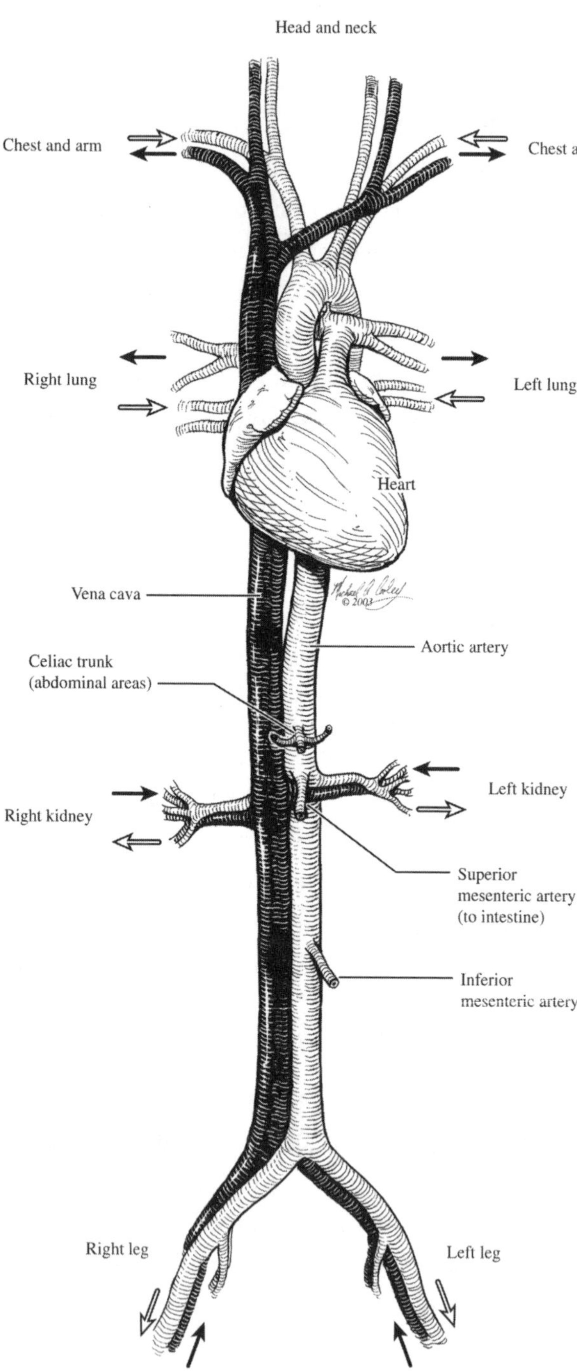

Fig. 2. The heart, with major arteries and veins. The arteries receive blood from the heart during ventricular contraction (the systolic phase). During relaxation of the heart and refilling of the ventricles, blood flows progressively into small arteries and ultimately into the capillaries (the diastolic phase).

pressure: During the relaxation phase of the heart, as blood flows into the ventricles, the pressure within the arteries reaches its lowest level, 80 mm Hg. Then, the heart contracts, sending a bolus of blood into the aorta, and, as a result, causes the pulse pressure to rise by 40, to 120. If the pulse pressure is decreased by 8.9 mm Hg, for instance, the work of the heart, mathematical manipulation reveals, has been decreased by 22 percent, which is an increment of considerable magnitude.

Establishing Parameters for Blood Pressure

The level of one's blood pressure is an important prognosticator of one's health. At the physician's office patients are nonplussed when the medical assistant approaches with a sphygmomanometer and stethoscope in hand. Determination of the blood pressure level is a routine office procedure.

What patients find is that the assistant who performs the assessment fails, with great regularity, to disclose the reading. And the attending physician often neglects to mention the subject. Patients want to know, and they expect a vital sign such as blood pressure to have parameters that define the normal and elevated levels with some degree of certitude. As the following section will show, however, any delineation must be set arbitrarily.

Blood Pressure, Stroke, and Heart Attack

It has long been recognized that high blood pressure is a risk factor for stroke (vascular accident involving the brain) and heart attack (obstruction of coronary artery flow to the contractile muscle

Table 1. Stroke and Heart Attack Events for Each Blood Pressure Bracket

	123/76	*136/84*	*148/91*	*162/99*	*175/105*
Number of Subjects	142,305	160,695	85,056	27,340	7,198
Stroke	151	243	213	136	100
Heart Attack	1,028	1,638	1,247	617	326

(From MacMahon, S et al. *The Lancet* 1990;**335**:765–774. Reproduced by permission from Elsevier)

fibers) and that the risk increases with the degree of blood pressure elevation. In 1990 a statistical analysis of long-term observational studies that had been published up to that time relating to the risk of high blood pressure were presented in *The Lancet*,[1] a prestigious medical publication of Great Britain. The report provided some much-needed information.

Nine major trials, involving a total of 422,594 individuals, were reviewed. Most were North American trials, but some were from Europe, Puerto Rico, and Hawaii. Each study was an event-rate determination of eight to ten years duration for stroke and heart attack.

Throughout the study period none of the subject-volunteers took antihypertensive medications. At entry, the blood pressure of each subject was determined. During the ensuing several-year period, the subjects were monitored for stroke, heart attack, or death. Following termination of the trials, the entire population was divided, for purpose of analysis, into five subgroups, depending on the severity of the initial blood pressure. The bracket for each ascending group, the number of subjects for each group, and the number of strokes/heart attacks for each group is shown in table 1.

Next, the relative risk of developing either stroke or heart attack was calculated for each blood pressure group and a plot was constructed (fig. 3). The horizontal axis shows the five ascending blood

Relative Risk of Stroke and of Heart Attack

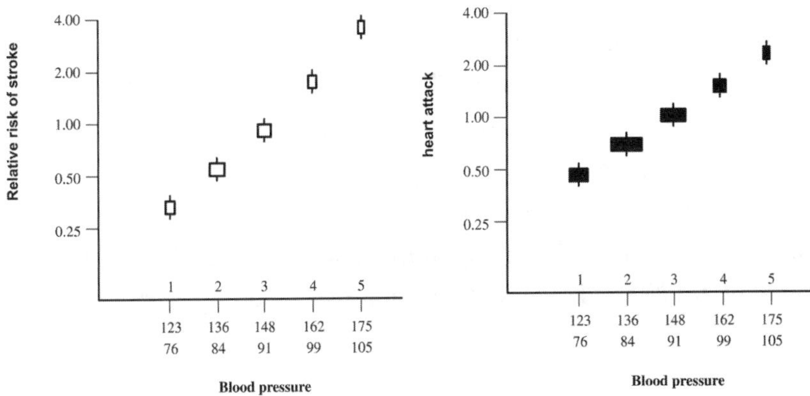

Fig. 3. Relative risk of developing stroke, on the left, and heart attack, on the right, with increase in blood pressure. The size of the boxes correspond to the number of events during the period of observation. The plot shows that the risk of developing either a stroke or a heart attack was directly related to the level of blood pressure throughout the normal and the hypertensive range.

The total number of strokes and heart attacks in the two lowest blood pressure brackets (123/76 and 136/84) was only slightly less than the total number for the three manifestly elevated blood pressure groups (148/91, 162/99, and 175/105). The risk of experiencing a stroke or heart attack is admittedly less when the blood pressure is at the lower levels. But there are many more people within the lower brackets. This is an important consideration in that a strategy which will have a major impact on the number of people experiencing stroke or heart attack must be directed at, and appropriately managed for, not only those with high blood pressure but also at those with lower blood pressure levels. (Reprinted with permission of *The Lancet* Ltd.)

pressure groups. The vertical axis projects the relative risk, in comparison to that for the entire group, for developing either stroke (on the left) or heart attack (on the right).

The plot showed that the risk of developing a stroke was *directly related to the level of blood pressure throughout the normal and the hypertensive range.* The same applied to heart attack, although the number of people dying from heart attack (represented by the size of the rectangular disc in the figure) was about four or five times greater than for stroke.

The risk of developing a stroke was fourteen (or so) times less for an individual with a normal blood pressure (118/72) than with a moderately raised blood pressure (172/105). The risk of heart attack was four times less.

The 1990 study showed that the risk of both stroke and heart attack develops not only among individuals in the high blood pressure range, of 140/90 and over, but also at lower blood pressure levels.

BLOOD VESSEL INJURY AS A RESULT OF HIGH BLOOD PRESSURE

The effects of high blood pressure can strike without warning. One dramatic development is blood vessel rupture, which, if it is in the brain, causes bleeding into the surrounding tissue (a hemorrhagic stroke). Less dramatically, high blood pressure can cause, over a period of many years, dilatation and weakening of the larger arteries (the aorta, particularly) within the body. Expansion by 40 percent is referred to as an *aneurysm*, which is susceptible to rupture if the blood pressure remains elevated.

Another target of high blood pressure is the heart. In order to perform the workload imposed by high blood pressure, the heart muscle thickens (the medical term for which is *hypertrophy*). Faced with the persistent challenge over several years, the heart, in time, begins to fail. As a result, the perfusion of arteries throughout the body becomes less and the function of the organs within the body is compromised.

High blood pressure takes its toll particularly on the smaller arteries (the so-called arterioles) in the body, especially those within the kidney, the brain, and the eye (fig. 4). The arterioles become thickened and narrowed (arteriosclerosis) as a result of the

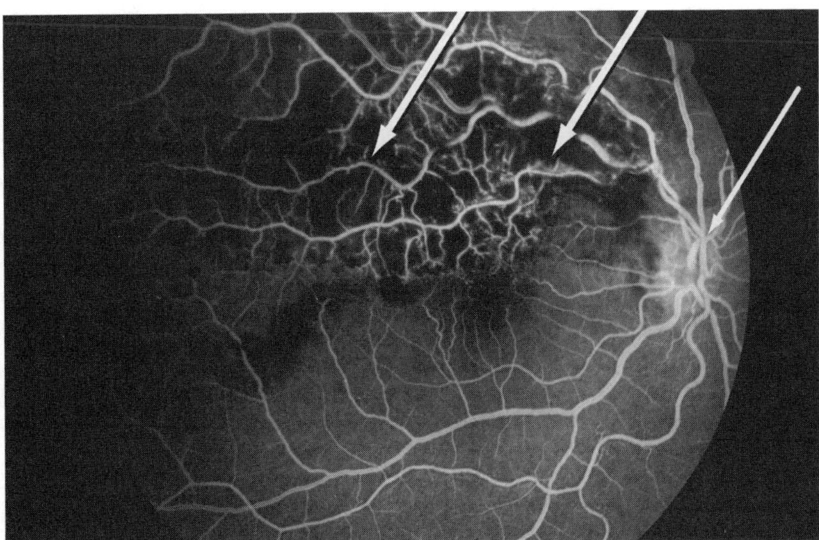

Fig. 4. Branch retinal vein occlusion, right eye. Sixty-two-year-old female, blood pressure 152/94. Circulation study (fluorescein angiogram). The obstruction has developed immediately superior to the nervehead (thin arrow) where an arteriole has compressed an underlying vein. The arteriole had become thickened (and hardened) as a result of long-standing high blood pressure. Flow has become stagnant secondary to the obstruction and capillaries have ruptured. A diffuse hemorrhage (broad arrows) extends through the superior and temporal portion of the retina. Visual acuity is reduced to 20/400.

persistent elevation in blood pressure. Constriction and occlusion can develop eventually.

Hypertensive sclerosis (hardening) of blood vessels within the brain hastens the onset of dementia, a condition that commences within one of four individuals by age eighty.

An early herald of dementia is the deterioration of cognition—that is, the ability to know, perceive, remember, imagine, think, reason, and judge. Cognition can be measured quantitatively with various psychometric tests. A study of 999 men seventy years of age and older, in Sweden, found that hypertension contributes significantly to the development of cognitive impairment.[2]

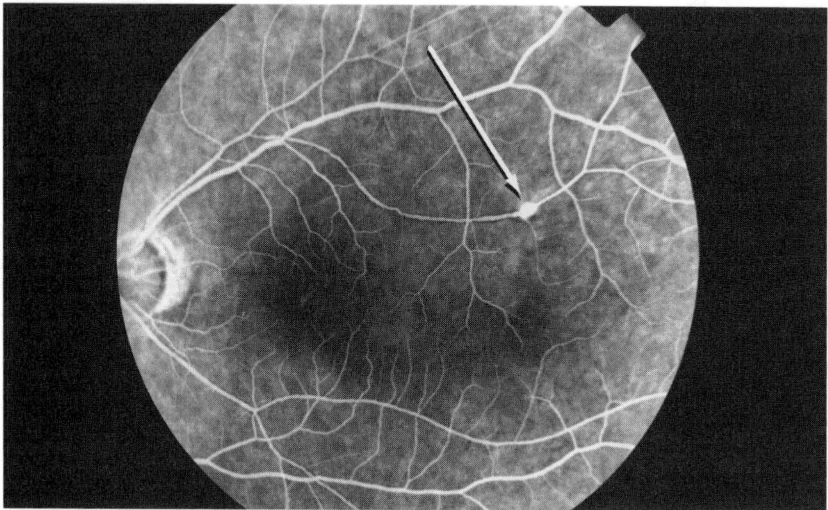

Fig. 5. Aneurysm (white/black arrow) of retinal arteriole with early hemorrhagic leakage (black speck along inferior margin of blood vessel). Male, fifty-eight years old. Blood pressure (BP) 145/90.

In another study that demonstrated an effect on cerebral function from high blood pressure, the intellectual capacity in untreated hypertensive men (diastolic blood pressure >105 mm Hg) showed impairment of vigilance and attention span in comparison to that of normotensive controls. And intellectual loss, measured over a ten-year period in still another study, was significantly greater in a group of patients with diastolic blood pressure >105 mm Hg when compared with matched normotensive controls.[3]

Damage to the arterioles of the kidney can impair nitrogen excretion so that hemodialysis can become necessary. In recent decades the requirement for such care has increased several times.

The effects of hypertension are observable within the retina of the eye. A not uncommon presentation for the retinal physician is hypertensive vein obstruction (fig. 4) or, with somewhat less frequency, a patient with complications ensuing from an arteriolar

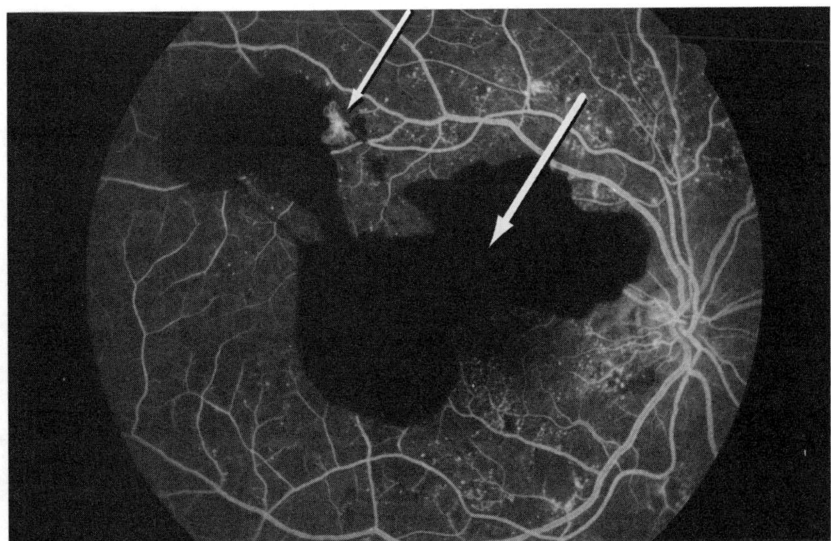

Fig. 6. Preretinal hemorrhage occurring in right eye of patient with diabetic retinopathy. Thirty-seven-year-old male, BP 142/100. Diabetes mellitus since age seventeen. Fluorescein circulation study. The white dots, the typical background finding of diabetic retinopathy, represent micro-size aneurysms of the retinal capillary system. The larger splotch (thin arrow) represents a proliferation of delicate and ill-formed blood vessels on the surface of the retina. Bleeding from the proliferation (broad arrow) commenced as the systemic blood pressure became progressively elevated. Visual acuity is only 5/400.

aneurysm (fig. 5). Of even greater concern for the eye is the deleterious effect that hypertension exerts on diabetic retinopathy (fig. 6) and age-related macular degeneration (fig. 7), the two leading causes of blindness within the industrialized countries of the world.

High Blood Pressure and Atherosclerosis

The larger arteries of the body are particularly susceptible to closure if the wall has been permeated by cholesterol, a condition termed *atherosclerosis*. In the early stage, the cholesterol deposit,

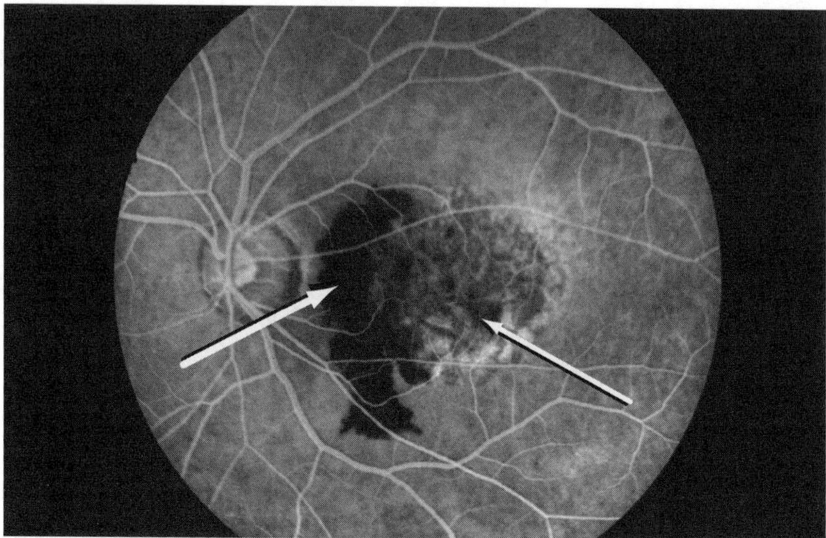

Fig. 7. Age-related macular degeneration with acute intraretinal hemorrhage (broad arrow), left eye. Seventy-year-old female, BP158/86. Visual acuity 20/200. New and ill-formed blood vessels (thin arrow) developed beneath the macula. The continuing effect of high blood pressure ultimately caused rupture of the abnormal blood vessels underlying the macular retina.

also termed *plaque*, has a fatty, gruel-like consistency, but in time an inflammatory response develops within the wall of the artery and a thin layer of scar tissue surrounds the plaque. High blood pressure increases the likelihood that the inner aspect of an atherosclerotic vessel will erode and tear (fig. 8). Cholesterol and fibrin debris released into the bloodstream from the rupture site travel further down the artery to a point where the lumen is smaller and the fragment clumps stop blood flow. Cellular death occurs within the distribution network of the obstructed vessel, a so-called ischemic, or infarcted, event. Often, a clot (a thrombosis) develops at the rupture site, too, to further intensify the degree of obstruction, or breaks loose and continues downstream (as an embolus) to obstruct a smaller vessel (fig. 9).

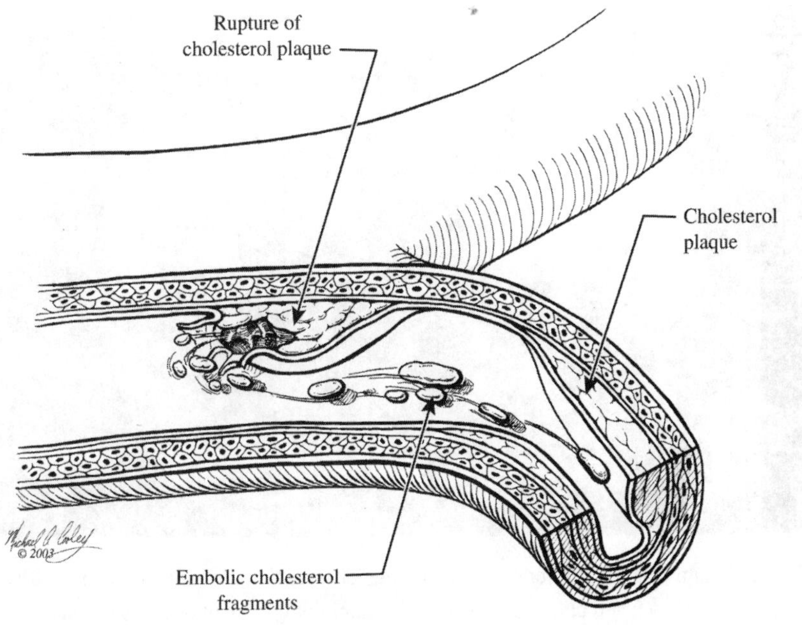

Fig. 8. Bifurcation of artery. Cross-sectional view of right side. Tear involving inner wall of artery releases cholesterol fragments into the bloodstream.

Cholesterol deposition within arterial walls is the result of the excessive intake of dietary fat. High blood pressure is the mechanism by which rupture/tear of the inner lining develops and blood vessel obstruction occurs.[4] The higher the blood pressure, the greater the sheer stress on the inner aspect of the arterial wall and the greater the likelihood of a breakdown involving a cholesterol deposit.

At What Point Should Blood Pressure Be Considered High?

For several decades hypertension has been defined in terms of 140/90. The 130–139 range is considered high-normal. Above

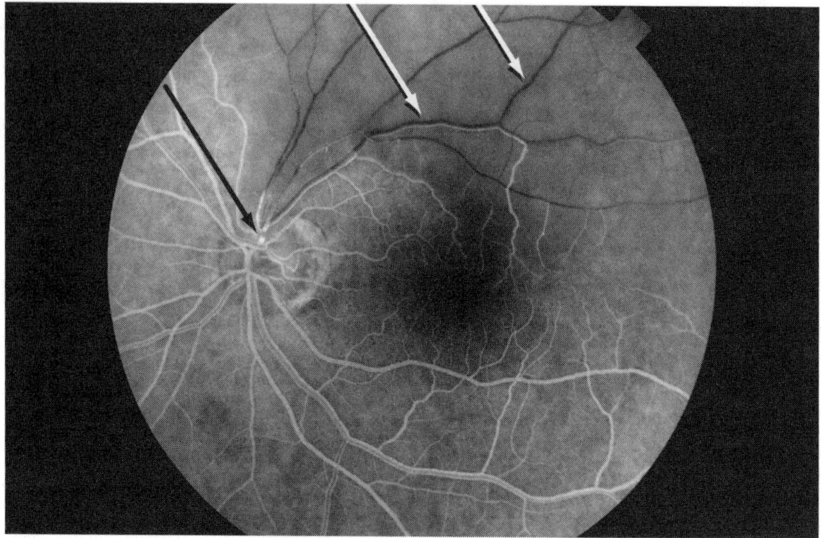

Fig. 9. Acute closure of arteriole within retina, left eye, sixty-three-year-old male, BP 147/84. Very slow filling of blood vessels within superior portion of retina (white/black arrows) as a result of cholesterol embolus (black arrow). Further studies led to identification of ulcerated plaque within aorta. Visual acuity 20/200.

140/90 is high. Doubt about how to define the 130–139 level became apparent in 1990 with the publication of the study in *The Lancet* and led to an analysis of data obtained from volunteers in Framingham, Massachusetts. That second study,[5] published in a November 2001 *New England Journal of Medicine* issue, involved several thousand volunteers and was coordinated by Boston-area medical institutions over a fourteen-year period.

The trial involved participants who at baseline examination could be classified into one of three nonhypertensive blood pressure categories: (1) ideal, less than 120/80 mm Hg, (2) normal, 120 to 129 systolic, and (3) high-normal, 130 to 139 systolic. Those with a systolic blood pressure above 140 were excluded.

The primary outcome of interest was the time to the occurrence

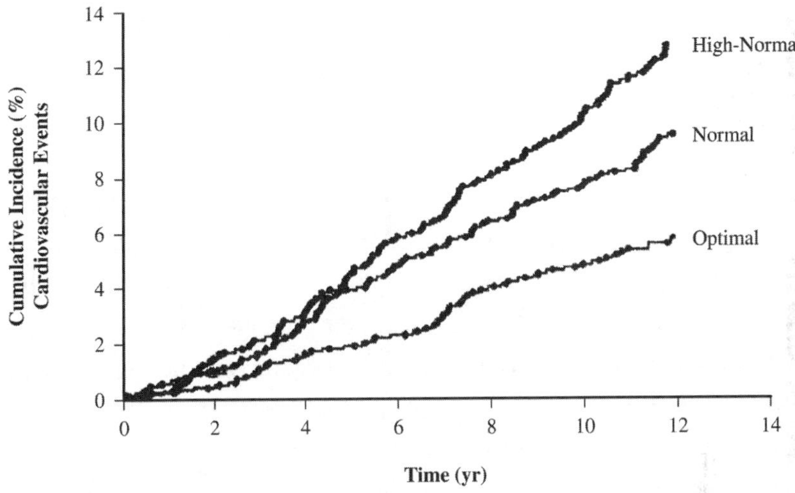

Fig. 10. Plotting the impact of high-normal blood pressure for men.[6] The plots show a progressively increasing incidence of cardiovascular events (stroke, heart attack, or congestive heart failure) over time for men with high-normal (a systolic pressure of 130–139 mm Hg), normal (120–129 mm Hg), and optimal (less than 119 mm Hg) blood pressure. High-normal is a pressure that cannot be casually dismissed. (Reproduced with permission from Vasan, RS et al. *New England Journal of Medicine* 2001;**345**:1291–1297 copyright 2001 Massachusetts Medical Society)

for a catastrophic blood vessel event, that is, stroke, heart attack, or congestive heart failure.

During the fourteen-year trial period, the catastrophic cardiovascular rate increased in a stepwise manner for each of the three blood pressure categories (fig. 10). High-normal (130–139 mm Hg) blood pressure was associated with a significantly greater risk of cardiovascular disease in both women and men. The findings serve as verification for the conclusion that many medical researchers had arrived at in recent years, namely: high-normal blood pressure (130–139 mm Hg) is more "high" than normal.

The importance of maintaining a low blood pressure becomes readily apparent from the Framingham study. One cannot be complacent with a systolic blood pressure in the 130–139 range.

REDUCING THE RISK OF STROKE/HEART ATTACK WITH A 8.9 MM HG REDUCTION IN BLOOD PRESSURE

Assume that the US adult population adhered to the 2001 DASH–1150 mg sodium diet and that a 8.9 mm Hg blood pressure reduction is achieved for each and every person. What would be the effect on the incidence of stroke and heart attack?

A statistician would provide an answer by reconstructing figure 3. He would simply shift plots, for stroke and heart attack, 8.9 units to the left. Essential to the mathematical calculation would be the numerical count for the five blood pressure groups, as shown in table 1.

As each group shifts to the left, the relative risk (size of the box) reduces by a considerable degree (fig. 11). By mathematical manipulation of that type, that is, a repeat calculation of the relative risk for each group, one comes to a percentage reduction of 46 percent for stroke and 32 percent for heart attack. It is fair to say, then, that an 8.9 mm Hg decrease in the blood pressure for the adult US population would produce a profound decrease in the incidence of stroke and heart attack.

A more complete characterization of blood pressure as a disease entity might show a stronger relationship than the data presented here. The important consideration is how many people are apt to adhere to a DASH–1150 mg sodium diet so that an 8.9 mm Hg reduction can be achieved. Not many. One problem is the high fat and sodium content of food served at fast-food outlets and of food consumed in the home, a problem that is the subject of the next chapter.

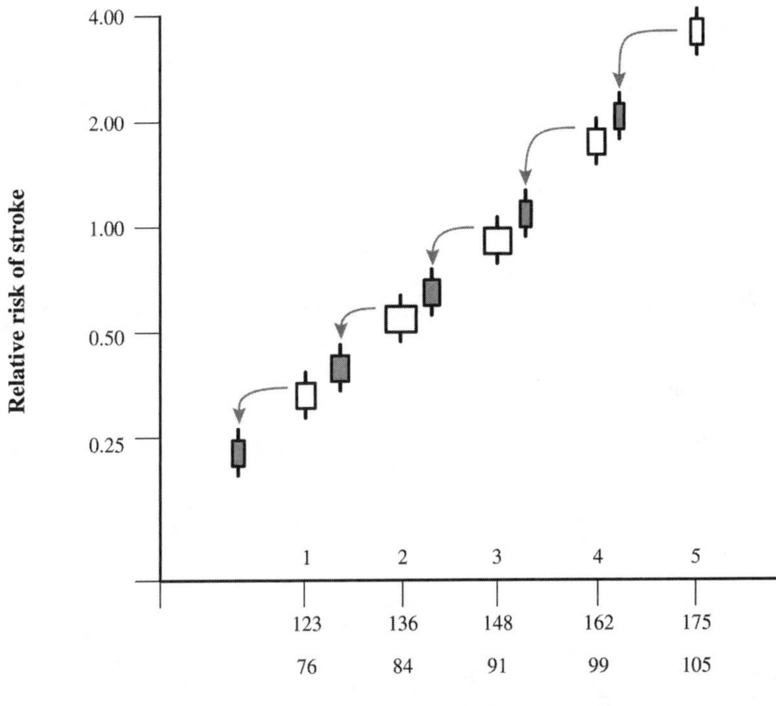

Fig. 11. Calculating the effect of a universal 8.9 mm Hg reduction in blood pressure. The number of strokes is adjusted as the blood pressure for each bracket is reduced by 8.9 mm Hg. Mathematical exercise of this type shows that the overall incidence of stroke would be reduced by 46 percent with adherence to the DASH–1150 mg sodium diet.

NOTES

1. MacMahon, S et al. Blood pressure, stroke, and coronary heart disease. *The Lancet* 1990;**335**:765–774.

2. Kilander, L et al. Hypertension is related to cognitive impairment. A 20-year follow-up of 999 men. *Hypertension* 1998;**31**:780–786.

3. Boller, F et al. Neuropsychologic correlates of hypertension. *Archives of Neurology* 1977;**34**:701

Wilke, F and Eisdorfor, C. Intelligence and blood pressure in the aged. *Science* 1971;**172**:959.

4. Many cardiovascular researchers believe that high blood pressure enhances the process by which cholesterol deposition occurs within the walls of arteries. Apparently, the increase in blood pressure promotes the transfer of cholesterol from the blood column through the inner lining of the artery.

5. Vasan, RS et al. Impact of high-normal blood pressure on the risk of cardiovascular disease. *New England Journal of Medicine* 2001; **345**:1291–1297.

6. The plot for women was similar but less steep.

CHAPTER 4

WHY THE CHALLENGE IS DIFFICULT

In their 2001 *New England Journal of Medicine* report, the DASH investigators noted that adherence to an enhanced fruit/vegetable, low-fat, and 1150 mg sodium diet would be a difficult undertaking for the US populace. This chapter will review why that is so.

For many years now dining out at fast-food outlets has been a popular American pastime. And at home, packaged items and processed foods are consumed more frequently than ever before. The DASH investigators expressed the concern that the general population is not aware of the high fat and salt content of either the fast-food outlets menu or of the processed items used in the home.

EATING OUT

To illustrate how difficult adherence to the DASH–1150 mg sodium diet can be, assume for an example day that one patronizes a fast-food outlet for each meal. Very few people do such a thing, although a truck driver might. The assumption is not unreasonable, though, since fast-food outlets are presently a dominant force in the American food chain. In 1970 Americans spent about $6 billion on fast food; in 2001 they spent more than $110 billion.[1] Three decades ago there was a handful of modest hot dog and hamburger stands in each city; presently, fast-food outlets have spread to every corner of the nation, selling a broad range of food wherever paying customers might be found. Fast food is now served at drive-throughs, airports, zoos, museums, high schools, elementary schools, Wal-Marts, gas stations, and even in hospital cafeterias.

Eric Schlosser, in *Fast Food Nation*, provided the following statistics: The typical American, he noted, now consumes approximately three hamburgers and four orders of french fries every week.

> Per capita consumption of ground beef is now about 30 pounds a year, with the vast majority consumed as hamburgers. A regular hamburger patty weighs 1.6 ounces: Using that [size] as a standard, Americans eat about 300 burgers a year or five to six a week.[2]

Mr. Schlosser went on to say that some patties are larger, a Quarter Pounder for instance. He adjusted his figures to come up with the approximation of three hamburgers a week.

For french fries, he noted that the per capita consumption of frozen potato products (a category that goes almost entirely into french fries) is about thirty pounds a year. A regular order at McDonald's weighs 68 grams. Converting the pounds to kilograms and then dividing that number by 68 leaves one with the number of french fry servings consumed annually by the US populace: 205, or about 4 per week.

Fast-food retail has achieved a high degree of popularity. To proceed in the paragraphs that follow with the assumption that a person patronizes a fast-food outlet for each meal during the day provides, at the very least, some insight regarding nutrient content of the US diet.

Assume that one patronizes a fast-food outlet for each meal during a representative day.

Breakfast is a stop at McDonald's on the way to work. The choices: biscuit with sausage and egg, hash browns with ketchup, coffee with milk and sugar.

Midmorning break is at Dunkin' Donuts: a plain donut.

Lunch is at Long John Silver's: two pieces of fish, coleslaw, fries, Diet Coke.

Evening meal is at Arby's: roast beef sandwich, salad with Thousand Island dressing, apple turnover, Diet Coke.

Table 1. Dining at Fast-Food Outlets[3]

Breakfast—McDonald's	*fat %*	*sodium (mg)*	*calories*
sausage biscuit with egg	60	1010	490
hash browns	55	330	130
ketchup, 1 packet	0	110	10
coffee with sugar and cream	85	4	44
Midmorning—Dunkin' Donuts[4]			
donut, plain	54	340	240
Lunch—Long John Silver's			
fish, 2 pieces	52	1400	460
coleslaw	41	310	170
french fries, regular size	52	500	250
Diet Coke, medium	0	40	0
Dinner—Arby's			
roast beef sandwich	44	1009	388
salad with Thousand Island dressing	90	420	260
apple turnover	38	180	330
Diet Coke, medium	0	40	0
Totals	**53%**	**5693 mg**	**2772 cal**

And what are the damages? As table 1 shows, the weighted average for fat content would be 53 percent, which is considerably higher than the 26 percent for the DASH diet. And the sodium content would be 5693 mg, or more than five times the goal of a 2001 DASH–1150 mg sodium diet.

EATING IN

In a second exercise, assume that meal preparation is done at home and that most of the items are packaged, frozen, or canned—that is, ready to go without much fuss and bother.

Table 2. Dining at Home—Processed Foods[5]

Breakfast	*fat %*	*sodium (mg)*	*calories*
Rice Krispies and 2% milk	12	381	180
Oscar Mayer bacon, 2 slices	77	290	70
wheat toast, 2 slices	13	295	137
butter	99	41	36
coffee with milk and sugar	85	4	44
Midmorning			
Lender's bagel, frozen, plain	5	320	150
Lunch			
turkey, 2 oz. Hormel Deli Petite	12	486	50
mustard, 1 tsp.	0	56	3
bread, 2 slices	13	295	137
potato chips	56	336	302
baked beans, 4 oz. Campbell's Homestyle	12	430	130
Coca-Cola	0	50	140
Dinner			
Red Barron pizza, 2 slices	51	1022	442
salad with Thousand Island dressing	90	420	260
breadsticks, 2	22	131	82
Totals	**45%**	**4557 mg**	**2163 cal**

At breakfast the menu might consist of cold cereal, milk, bacon, toast with butter, and coffee. At midmorning, a bagel. For lunch, assume: a turkey sandwich with mustard, potato chips, baked beans, and Coke. Finally, at dinner: pizza, salad with dressing, breadsticks, and tea.

The total for the at-home meals is shown in table 2. Again, the fat and sodium content of the 2001 DASH–1150 mg sodium diet has been exceeded by a considerable degree.

CEREAL

Breakfast cereals deserve extra comment. Rice Krispies, the food label for which is shown in figure 1, is an example of packaged cereals with a high salt content. The carbohydrate content is 29 grams. Rice Krispies contains no fat. But what about the 320 mg per serving sodium content?

Food labels can be helpful, but the true meaning of the salt content is often missed. One way to get a handle on this is to relate salt content of a particular item to that of ocean water. The author is indebted to Dr. Graham MacGregor for providing the following insight in his text *Salt, Diet and Health.*[6]

The salt (sodium and chloride) concentration of ocean water is 2.5 grams per 100 grams. To convert to sodium, one multiplies the weight of salt by 0.4. Thus, the sodium content for ocean water is 2.5 times 0.4, or 1.0 gram per 100 grams of water.

Return, next, to the Rice Krispies. The serving size is 33 grams. The sodium content is 320 mg. Assume that 4 ounces of milk are consumed with the cereal, another 62 mg of sodium. Sodium for the serving is 320 plus 62, or 382 mg.

An ounce weighs 28.35 grams. Therefore, the sodium concentration for a bowl of Rice Krispies is 382 mg per 5 ounces.

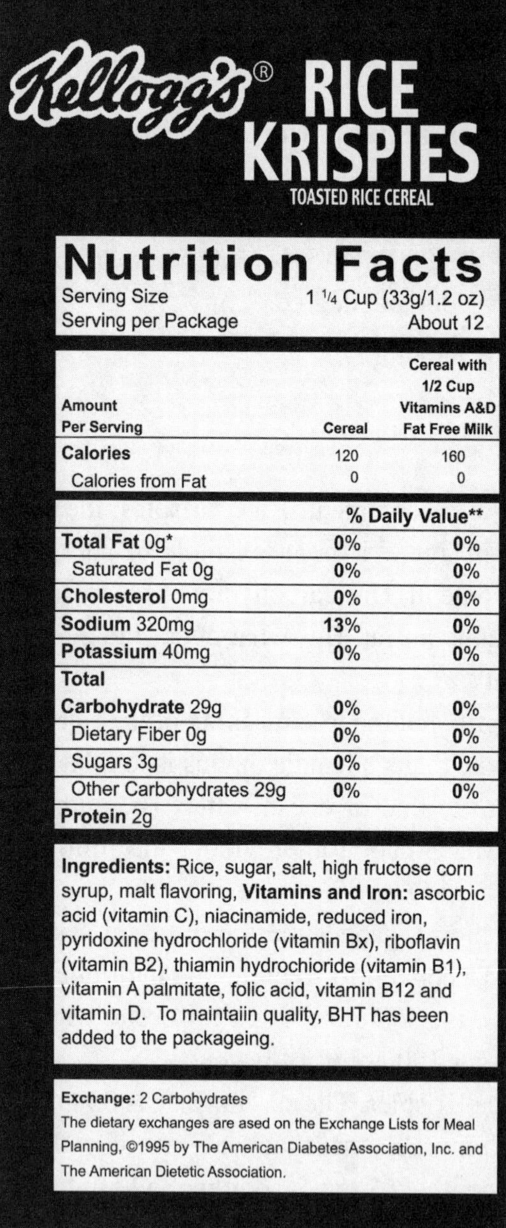

Kellogg's® RICE KRISPIES
TOASTED RICE CEREAL

Nutrition Facts

Serving Size 1 1/4 Cup (33g/1.2 oz)
Serving per Package About 12

Amount Per Serving	Cereal	Cereal with 1/2 Cup Vitamins A&D Fat Free Milk
Calories	120	160
Calories from Fat	0	0
		% Daily Value**
Total Fat 0g*	0%	0%
Saturated Fat 0g	0%	0%
Cholesterol 0mg	0%	0%
Sodium 320mg	13%	0%
Potassium 40mg	0%	0%
Total Carbohydrate 29g	0%	0%
Dietary Fiber 0g	0%	0%
Sugars 3g	0%	0%
Other Carbohydrates 29g	0%	0%
Protein 2g		

Ingredients: Rice, sugar, salt, high fructose corn syrup, malt flavoring, **Vitamins and Iron:** ascorbic acid (vitamin C), niacinamide, reduced iron, pyridoxine hydrochloride (vitamin Bx), riboflavin (vitamin B2), thiamin hydrochioride (vitamin B1), vitamin A palmitate, folic acid, vitamin B12 and vitamin D. To maintaiin quality, BHT has been added to the packageing.

Exchange: 2 Carbohydrates
The dietary exchanges are ased on the Exchange Lists for Meal Planning, ©1995 by The American Diabetes Association, Inc. and The American Dietetic Association.

Fig. 1. Current example of US food label, in this case for Rice Krispies. Amount of sodium, 320 mg per serving, is also expressed as a percentage (13%).[7]

Expressed otherwise, the sodium concentration is 382 mg per 146 grams, or, finally, 261 mg per 100 grams.

The above calculation shows that the sodium content for a bowl of Rice Krispies is 26 percent that of ocean water. Such a calculation causes considerable aggravation to the food industry, for they do not like the saltiness of their products compared to ocean water. Other popular cereal brands containing similar amounts of sodium are shown in table 3.

Why doesn't one realize that breakfast cereals are so salty while gulping down the contents in the morning? Many cereals contain added sugar. And

Table 3. High-Sodium Cereals

*Cereal**	*sodium* (mg)	*calories*
General Mills Cheerios	280	110
Hill Country Fare Corn Flakes	320	110
Kraft Post Toasties	278	107
General Mills Kix	270	120

*Adjusted to a 30 g serving weight[8]

on top of that it is customary to add a small amount of sugar to each serving. The sweetness provided by the added sugar is sufficient to disguise the salinity.

Fortunately, food manufacturers do offer cereals with low amounts of fat and salt. So the ultimate choice in the morning is clearly the responsibility of the consumer. Example cereals with low-fat and low-sodium content are shown in table 4.

PROCESSED AND PACKAGED FOODS

The problem with most canned and processed foods is that sodium in very large quantities is added during preparation, and potassium, a beneficial electrolyte, is removed.

Table 4. Low-Sodium Cereals

*Cereal**	*sodium* (mg)	*calories*
Skinners Raisin Bran	46	95
Quaker Puffed Rice	0	115
Kraft Post Shredded Wheat	0	100
Kellogg Kashi Go Lean	26	90

*Adjusted to a 30 g serving weight[9]

The electrolytic flip-flop that occurs when vegetables are canned is illustrated in table 5 for a ½ cup serving of two representative examples, green beans and corn. The calories for the fresh and the canned counterpart are essentially the same. Sodium, on the other hand, is increased many times during the canning process while potassium is decreased. For meats and cheese, the preparation for marketing produces much of the same—a sodium content that is much greater than the fresh counterpart and a potassium content that is lower. The contrast in electrolyte content for pork, beef, and milk and their processed counterparts is also shown in table 5.

Of course, sodium is added by the manufacturer during processing because of the perception that flavor and taste appeal is enhanced. But why is potassium reduced during that same process? Apparently, the perception among food processors is that *potassium adds a bitter note and there is a desire, therefore, to maintain potassium at a minimal level.*[10]

Table 5. Sodium and Potassium Content—Fresh vs. Processed Foods

Vegetable serving (1/2 cup)	*sodium* (mg)	*potassium* (mg)	*calories*
green beans (fresh)	3	115	17
green beans (canned), Del Monte	390	73*	20
corn (fresh)	11	208	66
corn (canned), Green Giant	345	158*	120
Meat serving	*sodium* (mg)	*potassium* (mg)	*calories*
pork (1 chop), fresh*	46	298	153
ham, Oscar Mayer, baked, 3 slices	782	168	65
beef (steak), fresh, 4 oz.*	64	408	152
bologna, Oscar Mayer, 2 slices	660	94	176
	sodium (mg)	*potassium* (mg)	*calories*
milk, whole, 1 cup	119	371	149
cheese, cheddar, 1 oz., Kraft	180	28*	120

*USDA National Nutrient Database[11]

FOOD LABELS

Since 1986 US food manufacturers have been required by Food and Drug Administration decree to include nutritional labeling on their products[12] (fig. 1). This action followed a strengthening of the view of medical practitioners and the public itself that dietary salt excess is a risk factor for the development of hypertension and other blood vessel complications.

In the years that have followed the FDA initiative, food labels have had only a marginal effect on consumer attitude, it would seem. The role of sodium chloride as a stimulator of taste receptors is well understood by food manufacturers. They are very aware that the average consumer is reluctant to sacrifice the flavor which salt adds to a product.

If the sodium content for a particular packaged food is reduced by 33 percent, the manufacturer is permitted to specify "less salt" or "reduced sodium" on the container. Here again flavor and product acceptability are the paramount issues.

For some products cost is an important factor in producing low- and reduced-sodium products. As a Campbell Soup Company representative admitted in 1986:[13] "To partly compensate for real and perceived loss of flavor in [reduced-salt] products, there is a necessity to add more ingredients, i.e., meat, vegetables, spices, and herbs. This adds substantially to the cost of those products."

The trade representative went on to say, in a report to *Food Technology* journal: "Finally, product development costs for low- and reduced-sodium products are considerably higher than for regular products. As a result, the large manpower and financial investment in developing viable low- and reduced-sodium products could become misspent resources, as scientific knowledge continues to evolve and alter the conventional wisdom over time." Actually, the accumulation of scientific knowledge since 1986, subsequent to Campbell's expressed concern regarding misspent resources, has indicated that more, and not less, product development cost should be allocated to low-salt foods.

Approximately 70 to 80 percent of the sodium intake is hidden in processed foods. When patients are advised to reduce dietary sodium, they will reluctantly remove the salt shaker from the table and, perhaps, reduce the amount of salt added to the cooking. But most are unaware of the very high sodium content of processed foods. The food-labeling program has been a big step forward in guiding the public toward better dietary choices. And in the future, one can anticipate that more, and not less, assistance of such type will be provided to the consumer.

THE CHALLENGE

The DASH Research Group questioned whether or not the US consumer is capable of challenging the fast-food giants and the food manufacturers. After all, food cultivation, processing, and dispersing is a two-trillion-dollar business, or one-third of the gross domestic product. On balance, though, the food industry is insignificant compared to what ordinary citizens can accomplish. Nobody in the United States is forced to patronize fast-food outlets or to purchase high-sodium processed foods. The first step for customers is by far the easiest: be selective. The executives in the food industry are not bad people. The performance of their business is their primary concern. They will sell fresh, wholesome, low-fat, and low-sodium food if the public so demands. They will sell whatever rings up a profit. The usefulness of the market, it's effectiveness as a tool, cuts both ways. The chief executive officers of Burger King, Kraft, Nabisco, and Pepsi/Frito-Lay should feel daunted. There are dozens of them, at most. The population of the United States, in comparison, is approaching three hundred million. A selective boycott, a refusal to buy, can speak much louder than words.

At the fast-food outlet, one should be aware of each and every ingredient. Either place an order or turn and walk out the door. In the grocery store, notice the ingredients, especially the sodium content. The consumer makes the choice. After all, it's the consumer's health that is at stake. Even in this era of quick service, consumers can have it their way.

Make comparisons. Reject items that do not measure up. The real power of the consumer is yet to be released.

NOTES

1. Schlosser, E. *Fast Food Nation*. New York: HarperCollins, 2002, p. 295.

2. Ibid.

3. For further information regarding specific items of particular fast-food merchandisers, consult their Web sites. They are required to post nutritional information since they dispense an identical product at each of their outlets.

Traditional restaurants and cafeterias have managed to escape governmental edicts. They have successfully argued that a customer will often request modification to or elimination of the condiments used during preparation. So electrolyte content might vary from one customer to the next. Cafeterias, on the other hand, have little room within which to make such an argument. The uncertainty one encounters with cafeteria food is whether or not a vegetable offered in the serving line is fresh or canned and whether or not a small, medium, or large amount of salt was used during its preparation. A requirement that nutritional information be posted for each item would not be an unreasonable burden for management.

4. "Jumpin' Jelly! Doughnuts Dominate Dining Growth" read the

headline in the May 27, 2003, Money section of *USA Today*. "Krispy Kreme plans to add 77 stores next year," the article by Bruce Horowitz went on to say. "In June, it will open its first store in Australia and later this year, in the United Kingdom." As for the leading chain, Dunkin' Donuts, it planned to open three hundred stores during the next year. One industry spokesman explained the present-day popularity of doughnuts this way: "People are so health conscious that doughnuts are a fun splurge." A fun splurge?

5. Manufacturer's food label information.

6. MacGregor, G and de Wardener, H. *Salt, Diet and Health*. Cambridge: Cambridge University Press, 2000, p. 223.

7. See paper by Darnaif, G and Khoo, C. Developing low- and reduced-sodium products: an industrial perspective. *Food Technology* 1986;**40(12)**:105–107.

8. Manufacturer's food label information.

9. Manufacturer's food label information.

10. See paper by Darnaif, G and Khoo, C. Developing low- and reduced-sodium products: an industrial perspective. *Food Technology* 1986;**40(12)**:105–107.

11. For some items electrolyte concentration was obtained from http://www.nal.usda.gov/fnic/cgi-in/nut_search.pl.

12. Heimbach, J. The growing impact of sodium labeling of foods. *Food Technology* 1986;**40(12)**:102–104.

13. Ibid.

CHAPTER 5

THE SALT PRODUCERS

Unseemly has been the response of the US and Canadian salt producers—American Rock Salt Company, the Canadian Salt Company Ltd., Cargill Salt, Exportadora de Sal, S.A. de C.V., Lyons Salt Company, Morton Salt Division, North American Salt, Sifto Canada Inc., and United Salt Corporation—to the published reports that document untoward health effects resulting from the excessive use of dietary salt. Their official statements, orchestrated through a public relations agency known as the Salt Institute,[1] have rejected each and every medical study documenting an adverse effect to dietary salt. Their pro-salt stance is similar to that waged by the tobacco industry years ago. But, though we need not smoke, we have to eat, and as life becomes more hectic and less domesticated, there is an increasing dependency on readily available foods that can be quickly prepared. The demand for processed foods can only be expected to increase.

Equally defensive are the food manufacturers who with

increasing frequency counter adverse medical reports with public relations campaigns. The entire food industry is well aware of the medical trials pertaining to salt usage. To date, no course of action has been offered by either the salt producers or the food industry regarding what remedies should be taken.

SALT INSTITUTE

Much of the defensive effort has been channeled through the Salt Institute, the promotional arm for the thirty-two-member association of salt producers (fig. 1). Although the evidence that the current level of salt intake has harmful effects is now very powerful, the Salt Institute has dispersed the opposing viewpoint with no small effect. Its activities have been previously reviewed by G. A.

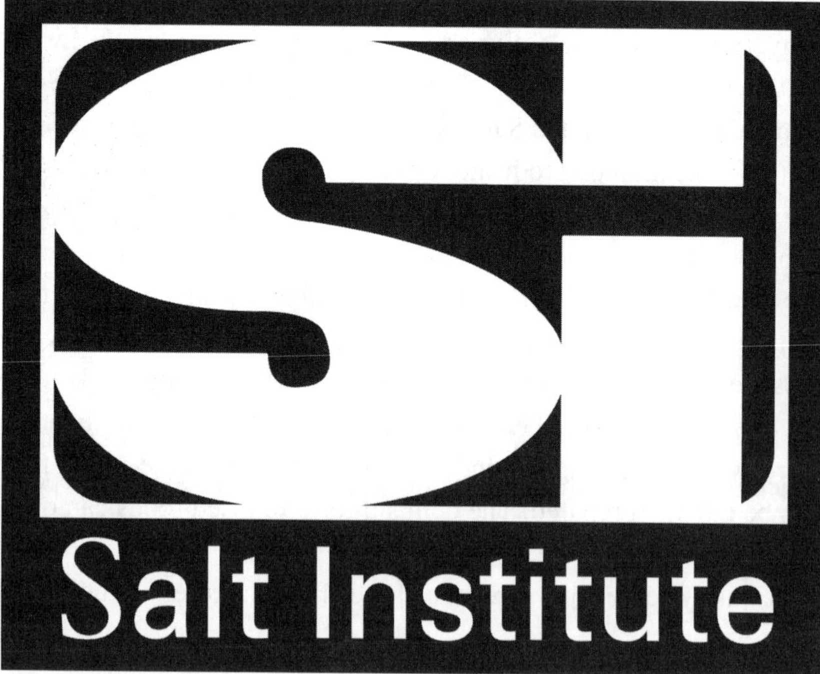

Fig. 1. Logo for the Salt Institute.

MacGregor and H. E. de Wardener, professors of medicine at the University of London, in their text *Salt, Diet and Health*.[2] For this chapter, I have drawn from a section in their book titled "The Industrial Conspiracy" and have added new material of my own.

The material released by the Salt Institute can be accessed through its Web site, www.saltinstitute.org. Its position in regard to health concerns attributed to dietary salt is unabashedly prejudiced. Often, its statements are unsupported by fact, such as: "Most humans tolerate a wide range of dietary intake, from about 250 mg/day to over 30,000 mg/day."[3] Actually, the lower limit for sodium is considerably less than 250 mg. Dr. Walter Kempner at Duke University Medical School routinely managed some of his patients with a sodium dietary regimen of 50 mg daily. In regard to the 30,000 mg upper limit for sodium, which the Salt Institute claims can be tolerated without ill effect, a search of the medical literature of the past fifty years failed to uncover a medical report that substantiates such an upper limit. No matter. The 2001 DASH study showed that a much less amount, that is, 3500 mg, is associated with an increase in blood pressure.

The Salt Institute has also stated, on its Web site, that the "blood pressure for most people is only marginally effected by sodium dietary intake up to the 7,000–11,500 mg range." That remark is also off the mark. Most of the trials that have been reported during the past fifty years indicate the opposite. Blood pressure is directly related to sodium intake throughout the low, normal, and high ranges of dietary sodium intake.

One would think that as an information agency for the salt manufacturers, the Salt Institute would disseminate all medical reports pertaining to salt and health regardless of the results or outcome. No chance. Instead, its position is so entrenched that an observer, impartial or otherwise, surely questions whether the obvious conflict of interest has impaired the institute's judgment. At times, the audacity of its opinion has led to awkward and embarrassing positions.

INTERSALT

During the past fifteen years the Salt Institute has carried out a tireless campaign to discredit the results of an internationally supervised study known as INTERSALT. That study, sponsored by eleven international medical agencies, combined the efforts of ninety-two investigators in fifty-two population centers within thirty-two countries. The results were published in a 1988 issue of the *British Medical Journal* (*BMJ*).[4]

For each of the 10,074 volunteer subjects, the research team determined (1) sitting-position blood pressure and (2) twenty-four-hour urinary excretion of sodium. Compilation of that data revealed a strong correlation between urinary sodium excretion, which is, essentially, equal to the dietary intake of sodium during the same twenty-four-hour period, and blood pressure. The study further showed that a sodium reduction of 2300 mg per day could, in adults, decrease systolic blood pressure by 9 mm Hg. The result is of similar magnitude to the 6.7 mm Hg reduction reported by the DASH researchers for the typical USA dietary group in their 2001 report.[5]

The Salt Institute, in its self-proclaimed role as the "world's foremost source of authoritative information about salt," viewed the *BMJ* INTERSALT study with skepticism. It raised several objections to the *BMJ* editors and requested that the INTERSALT investigators reanalyze the data using statistical methodology suggested by the institute.[6]

The second analysis again showed a significant relationship between salt intake and blood pressure. That information was made available by the INTERSALT investigators to the Salt Institute in 1994.

Uproar

The Salt Institute set aside the requested reevaluation and, in time, submitted for publication analyses of its own. That material was accepted by the *BMJ* and, in 1996, the institute's analysis/interpretation of the INTERSALT data was published.[7]

In that same issue, the *BMJ* published additional statistical analyses that had been independently performed at the behest of the INTERSALT investigators. The editorial commentary that introduced the subject for *BMJ* readers began: "INTERSALT findings confirmed and strengthened."[8]

The analytical review, by researcher Malcolm Law, professor of environmental and preventive medicine, Royal London School of Medicine, was a confirmation of the original INTERSALT data.[9] He found the mathematical methodology that had been employed originally to be above reproach and wrote a piece titled "Commentary: Evidence on Salt Is Consistent" to that effect.[10] The *BMJ* editors published his remarks immediately succeeding the Salt Institute submission.

The *BMJ* editorial reported the controversy:

> The Salt Institute can be seen at work on p. 1283, using data from the INTERSALT study to try to discredit it. We publish this analysis not because we believe it[11] but so as to present readers with an example of how the salt industry works. The Institute's paper is followed by two stinging commentaries. Readers will make up their own minds.[12]

A second editorial[13] in the May 18, 1996, issue of the *BMJ* elaborated further under the rebuking title "The Food Industry Fights for Salt":

> Like any group with vested interests, the food industry resists regulation. Faced with a growing consensus that salt increases blood pressure and the fact that 65–85% of dietary salt comes from processed foods, some of the world's major food manufacturers have adopted desperate measures to try to stop governments from recommending salt reduction. Rather than reformulating their products, manufacturers have lobbied governments, refused to cooperate with expert working parties, encouraged misinformation campaigns, and tried to discredit the evidence. This week's *BMJ* finds them defending their interests as vigorously as ever.

The editorial continued:

> The Salt Institute's letter is the latest volley in a 20-year campaign by the food industry, waged since the role of diet in heart disease became a public health issue. The aim is to promote the view that data from population studies have little bearing on individual patients and, in the case of salt, no basis in human physiology.

And concluded:

> The food industry has everything to gain from keeping the controversy alive. Common salt is the main source of flavour in processed foods. Tasting panels show that low salt foods are often unappetizing and there is currently no good alternative to sodium chloride. Improving flavour by adding more natural ingredients (such as fruit and vegetables) would be expensive.

Jeremiah Stamler, MD, professor in the Department of Preventive Medicine, Northwestern Medical School, Chicago, was the author of the INTERSALT reply to the Salt Institute's piece.[14] His comments included the following statements:

> The Salt Institute continues to misrepresent the findings of INTERSALT (and other studies) on salt and blood pressure. . . . Not only does the Salt Institute misrepresent or omit INTERSALT findings showing higher salt intake is related to higher individual blood pressure and greater slope of blood pressure with age; it also chooses to ignore data—accumulated over decades by countless other studies, with every method of investigation—that have found the same relation.

Since the 1996 INTERSALT controversy, few medical researchers, it appears, have paid much attention to the statements emanating from the Salt Institute. Its efforts to disparage INTERSALT have not ceased, however. The INTERSALT study, the Salt Institute continues to maintain, is "controversial."[15] If INTERSALT has been accepted by the medical profession, one is entitled to ask, to whom is the study controversial?

Salt Institute's Position in Regard to the DASH Research Group Studies

Consider the response of the Salt Institute to the DASH studies. Initially, the 1997 DASH trial was described in the Salt Institute position statements as a "high mineral diet" as though there is something undesirable about the amount of potassium, magnesium, and calcium provided by a diet with enhanced fruits and vegetables and low-fat dairy products. Later, that designation was abandoned. Perhaps they realized, on review, that the additional potassium, magnesium, and calcium provided by the DASH diet amounts to only 1500 mg, or so.

When the DASH–1150 mg sodium study was published in 2001, the salt manufacturers were on the attack again. They stated that the trial showed "scant additional benefit (in blood pressure) to a massive reduction in dietary sodium." Later they insisted that the information provided by the trial applies only to "salt-sensitive" individuals.[16]

WORLD HEALTH ORGANIZATION (WHO)

In early 2002 the Salt Institute[17] was asked by WHO to respond to the draft of a report, "Diet, Nutrition, and the Prevention of Chronic Diseases," prior to the fifty-fifth World Health Assembly in Geneva. In the statement that followed, the Salt Institute criticized a proposal that would lower the recommended daily sodium intake from 3500 to 2000 mg. The institute's statement minimized the DASH–1150 mg sodium study, among other protestations, and contended, generally speaking, that dietary sodium reduction had no "basis in science," which is to say that dietary sodium reduction is not established by rigorous scientific data. The Salt Institute went on to contend that the causative mechanism for cardiovascular, diabetic, and osteoporotic disease, each of which was considered separately in its statement to WHO, had not been sufficiently elucidated in the research studies to justify the proposed 2000 mg dietary sodium recommendation.

WHO was not deterred by the Salt Institute's protestations. In early 2003 it officially recommended a maximum nutrient goal of 2000 mg for sodium.[18] Hanneman of the Salt Institute did not concede defeat. By May of 2004 he had resumed his attack on WHO with Dr. Muhammed Nasir Khan, president of the World Health Assembly.[19]

AMERICAN PUBLIC HEALTH ASSOCIATION

The efforts of the Salt Institute are unceasing. In 2002 it took aim at the American Public Health Association (APHA). The latter is the largest public health organization, representing more than fifty thousand members from over fifty public health occupations.[20]

In a policy statement the APHA had urged the restaurant and food-processing industries to dramatically lower the amount of sodium consumed by Americans. "America is hooked on snacks and foods high in sodium," said Mohammad N. Akhter, MD, then executive director of the APHA.[21] "The bad news is this diet is killing us. The good news is we can prevent this from happening by making changes in our food supply and by making wise food choices through better understanding of food labels."

Stephen Havas, MD, professor of epidemiology and preventive medicine at the University of Maryland School of Medicine and lead author of the APHA policy, went on to say, "Americans are consuming an ever increasing amount of processed foods high in sodium at home, at work, at school, and in restaurants." "Most consumers are unaware that these foods are loaded with sodium," added Havas. "The excess sodium in these foods is unnecessary and leads to a large, preventable toll of hypertension, premature death, and disability. Implementation of this policy [the APHA policy, adopted at the November 2002 annual meeting in Philadelphia, calls for a 50 percent reduction of the sodium content in processed foods over the next ten years] by the food-processing and restaurant industries could potentially save approximately 150,000 lives annually."

The Salt Institute immediately challenged the APHA with comments of its own.[22] "If you had told me," said Richard L. Hanneman, president of the Salt Institute, "that public officials had made this recommendation 25 years ago, or even 20 years ago, I could understand it, even though I'd respond that they (the APHA) should wait for the evidence to come in. That's what many scientists thought then." Hanneman went on to dampen the concerns about salt by explaining that "the problem is 'salt sensitivity' not 'salt intake.'"

In other words, Hanneman's position is that there are certain people, perhaps, who are sensitive to salt. These people, presumably, should restrict the amount of salt in their diet. But salt restriction should not, and need not, apply to everyone.

What Hanneman refuses to acknowledge is this: While some people do show a greater blood pressure response to dietary salt than others, the response is universal to some degree or another for the entire population. No one is excluded.

Hanneman also went on to explain: "The solution to [any US dietary problem] is not less salt, but more fruits, vegetables, and low-fat dairy products." Four years earlier such a diet had been belittled by the Salt Institute as being "high mineral."

M. H. ALDERMAN, MD, A SALT INSTITUTE ALLY

Dr. M. H. Alderman, professor of medicine at Albert Einstein Medical School in New York, requires some words of comment. He has been a persistent critic of studies which show that salt adversely affects one's health and has published information that advances the opposing point of view. Dr. Alderman consults with and attends meetings of the Salt Institute.

A 1995 paper of Alderman's made the extraordinary inference in the journal *Hypertension*[23] that a habitual reduction in dietary salt increased the risk of heart attack. That deduction was based on an unfortunate interpretative blunder as subsequent correspondence within the same journal pointed out. Alderman and associates had assumed, for a group of analyzed patients, that the salt intake following a five-day reduction phase represented habitual intake.[24] As Cook, Cutter, and Henneckens pointed out in their critique of the study, it was unjustified to assume that an individual's salt intake on the fifth day of an imposed low-salt diet reflects an individual's habitual intake of salt.[25]

The Alderman report was accepted without reservation by the Salt Institute and used, shortly thereafter, in a Citizen's Petition to the US Food and Drug Administration.[26] The petition alleged that there are safety considerations associated with the restriction of salt. Later, the Food and Drug Administration stated, after hearing many representations, "No conflicting evidence has been presented" to demonstrate that a moderate but significant reduction in salt intake would have any adverse health effect.

This embarrassing episode has received no comment from the Salt Institute. Dr. Alderman's 1995 publication continues to be highlighted by the Salt Institute in its policy statements.

Later, in 1998, Dr. Alderman published another study, which was purported to show an inverse relationship between sodium intake and cardiovascular morbidity.[27] The Salt Institute spared no expense in paying respect to the results of the study, and continues to do so. The only trouble is that the results have been contested. When the total caloric intake is properly adjusted for the subjects of the study, according to Dr. F. Sacks in a May 2002 issue of the *New England Journal of Medicine*,[28] the results reported by Alderman become reversed. That is, the cardiovascular death rates are higher (as one would expect) when the sodium intake is higher.

Conflicts of Interest

Until the last decade or so, it was thought that integrity was just built into the fabric of medical science. In recent years it has become evident that observational studies are open to bias, apparent or otherwise. Such a state of affairs surely exists with the studies relating to dietary salt. In the end, the researchers will surely get it right. Science is based on cold facts that can be quantified and reproduced and subjected to rigorous testing. Science is rapidly becoming the foundation of medicine. The art of medicine, of former times, is based on impressions and subjective experiences that often can be neither clearly defined nor accurately quantified. The Salt Institute would do itself a favor by stepping back from the fray that goes on between medical researchers and accept only evidence-based truths. At this point its rhetoric dishonors the entire field of study.

FOOD TECHNOLOGY

According to the *Chemical and Engineering News*,[29] Federal Drug Administration regulations permit a food processor to add to food substantially any amount of sodium chloride. The food processors add salt in excess of that provided by nature to improve the so-called taste of the product. This is an effort to produce something from a can or package that is tangy, palatable, and attractive. Food processors cannot be blamed for chemical additions that increase sales. But there is an obligation to provide a nutritious product. Consumers will be more and more demanding in the information age in which we now live. The Salt Institute, the food manufacturers, and the fast-food industry had better beware.

LITIGATION

Some activists are plotting strategies to bring lawsuits against the food industry with tactics similar to those of the antitobacco lobbyists. So far, the fast-food industry has borne the brunt of the attack. In July 2002, a 272-pound New York City man sued four fast-food chains, alleging that their food contributed to his obesity, heart disease, and diabetes. Three months later, in October, parents of two New York teenagers sued McDonald's claiming Big Macs made their children obese.[30] In a brief statement the National Restaurant Association called the lawsuit "senseless, baseless, and ridiculous."

Food manufacturers are concerned that litigation could be used against them, too. Even though consumers do not consistently make nutritious and healthy food choices, the manufacturers feel the threat of litigation and have become alarmed.

The Salt Institute has stated that the primary risk causing high blood pressure is "beyond our control, since we can't choose our parents." "Genetic factors," it notes, "explain a quarter to half of blood pressure variability" and "five times more than stress, physical activity/exercise, smoking, and of course, diet." How easy it is to blame our genes and, by doing so, be resigned to the cravings of our appetites rather than to make the necessary dietary choices and protect our health. The fallback on genes will not work in the new millennium. People are beginning to realize that there are other explanations, and they will insist that the Salt Institute provide impartial information or, otherwise, be subject to litigation.

NOTES

1. The Salt Institute also includes several worldwide salt producers within its associate membership. See its Web site: http://www.saltinstitute.org.

2. MacGregor, GA and de Wardener, HE. The industrial conspiracy. In: *Salt, Diet and Health.* MacGregor and de Wardener (eds.). Cambridge: Cambridge University Press, 1998.

3. http://www.saltinstitute.org.

4. INTERSALT Cooperative Research Group. INTERSALT: an international study of electrolyte excretion and blood pressure. Results for 24-hour urinary sodium and potassium. *British Medical Journal* 1988; **297**:319–328. The work was launched under the auspices of the Council

on Epidemiology and Prevention of the International Society and Federation of Cardiology (ISFC) and was supported by grants from the Wellcome Trust (United Kingdom); the National Heart, Lung, and Blood Institute (United States); the International Society of Hypertension; the World Health Organization; the Heart Foundations of Canada, Great Britain, Japan, and the Netherlands; the Chicago Health Research Foundation; the FWGO-FMRS (Belgian National Research Foundation), and the ASLK-CGER (Parastatal Insurance Co., Brussels).

5. For the 2001 DASH-sodium trial, the DASH Research Group purposely set the sodium restriction at 100 mmol, or 2300 mg. That increment allows for easy comparison from one trial to another.

6. MacGregor, GA and de Wardener, HE. The industrial conspiracy. In: *Salt, Diet and Health.* MacGregor and de Wardener (eds.). Cambridge: Cambridge University Press, 1998.

7. Hanneman, RL. INTERSALT: hypertension rise with age revisited. *British Medical Journal* 1996;**312**:1283–1284.

8. Editorial staff. INTERSALT findings confirmed and strengthened. *British Medical Journal* 1996;**312**:1238.

9. Law, M. Commentary: evidence on salt is correct. *British Medical Journal* 1996;**312**:1285–1287.

10. Professor Law explained how reanalysis of the INTERSALT data with elimination of some centers, as proposed by R. L. Hanneman, president of the Salt Institute, made no difference. He went on to say: "Not surprisingly the US Salt Institute, the organization representing the salt producers, disagrees. Its response enshrouds the salt issue in confusion . . . and, [Hanneman's paper] on these data is so opaque that it obfuscates rather than elucidates. Later, Law concludes, additional study only confirms the suspicion that this [Hanneman's submission to the *British Medical Journal*] is not a competent analysis." Law's final statement was particularly bitter: "This analysis [Hanneman's] is of service only to illustrate the length to which a commercial group will go to protect its market when presented with clear evidence detrimental to its interest."

11. As Professors MacGregor and de Wardener explained on page 205 of their text: The key reason for the Salt Institute's different interpre-

tation of the data was that in doing its sums it had not standardized for age and sex and had not adjusted for body weight and alcohol intake.

12. Editorial staff. INTERSALT findings confirmed and strengthened. *British Medical Journal* 1996;**312**:1238.

13. Ibid.

14. Stamler, J et al. Commentary: sodium and blood pressure in the INTERSALT study and other studies—in reply to the Salt Institute. *British Medical Journal* 1996;**312**:1285–1287.

15. http://www.saltinstitute.org/pubstat/nhbpepcc.html.

16. http://www.saltinstitute.org/pubstat/fnb.html.

17. http://www.saltinstitute.org/pubstat/who-4-02.html.

18. http://www.who.int/hpr/doc/who_fao_expert_rep.

19. http://www.saltinstitute.org/pubstat/who-5-18-04.html.

20. http://www.apha.org/about.

21. http://www.apha.org/news/page/2002/sodium_consumption.html.

22. http://www.saltinstitute.org/pubstat/ (November 12, 2002) Richard Hanneman, president, Salt Institute.

23. Alderman, ML et al. Low urinary sodium is associated with greater risk of myocardial infarction among treated men. *Hypertension* 1995;**25**:1144–1152.

24. See Professors MacGregor and de Wardener's characterization of the 1995 Alderman paper on page 210 of their book, to wit, "It is embarrassing to have to point out the translucent fallacy of this heady extrapolation. It was totally unjustified."

25. Cook, NR and Cutter, JA and Henneckens, CH. Editorial comments. An unexpected result for sodium—causal or casual? *Hypertension* 1995;**25**:1153–1154.

26. MacGregor, GA and de Wardener, HE. The industrial conspiracy. In: *Salt, Diet and Health*. MacGregor and de Wardener (eds.). Cambridge: Cambridge University Press, 1998.

27. Alderman, MH et al. Dietary sodium intake and mortality: the National Health and Nutritional Examination Study (NHANES 1). *The Lancet* 1998;**351**:781–785.

28. Sacks, FM et al. Correspondence. *New England Journal of Medicine* 2001;**344**:1718.

29. Riddick, TM. *Control of Colloid Stability through Zeta Potential.* Wynnewood, PA: Livingston Publishing Company, 1968, p. 198.

30. Kever, J and Fergus, MA. A childhood epidemic. *Houston Chronicle*. October 6, 2002, pp. 1 and 16A.

CHAPTER 6

THIRST

What has become firmly established by medical researchers is the effect dietary salt has on the sensation of thirst. Initially, animal studies[1] in 1953, 1955, and 1963 showed a predictable thirst response to intentional dietary salt loading. In the 1980s the animal studies were further refined and the relationship was found to be strong and reproducible.[2] Next, studies at St. George's Hospital Medical School in London by Feng He and others confirmed a similar relationship for humans.[3] Professors Feng He, G. A. MacGregor, and their associates performed two groundbreaking trials that defined the quantitative effect of dietary salt intake on thirst.

First, in an experimental study, subjects with elevated blood pressure who had not had previous pharmaceutical treatment or in whom treatment had been stopped for at least three months were fed a high-sodium diet of approximately 6000 mg/day and then, on the fifth day, the diet was switched to a low-sodium intake of 350 mg/day. The subjects (104 in number) were permitted free access to water. At the end of each dietary period, twenty-four-hour urine samples were measured for volume and sodium content.

In most temperate climates the body needs about a liter of fluid a day. If, however, the consumption of sodium is increased, the sodium concentration of the blood will rise, a process that stimulates thirst and the amount of fluid one drinks. As the St. George's Hospital Medical School's experiments demonstrated, the relationship also works in reverse. When the subjects were switched from the high- to the low-sodium diet, urinary volume decreased by 0.9 liters (or one quart, approximately) and urinary sodium by 5900 mg (fig. 1). The plot of all the intercepts showed that urinary volume decreased by 160 ml for a 1000 mg reduction in sodium excretion (fig. 2).

In a temperate climate the amount of water loss in perspiration is negligible, so urine volume was a true reflection of thirst and water intake.

Next, Professor He and his associates looked at the sodium intake/urinary volume relationship in a somewhat different kind of study, an observational analysis. They recruited 637 patients with mild, untreated hypertension and asked them to continue their normal diet while collecting twenty-four-hour urine samples for volume and sodium measurement. From that information they were able to plot twenty-four-hour urine volume against twenty-four-hour urine sodium as had been done in the initial, experimental study. A 1000 mg/day reduction in sodium intake caused a 150 ml decrease in twenty-four-hour volume. The plot of that relationship is shown in figure 3. The regression lines for both the experimental and the observational studies were quite similar.

Finally, when He and MacGregor superimposed their data on the results from the INTERSALT study of 1988, each regression line was found to be very similar (also shown in fig. 3).[4] The consistent data between the experimental and observational studies and the INTERSALT studies demonstrate that salt intake is an impor-

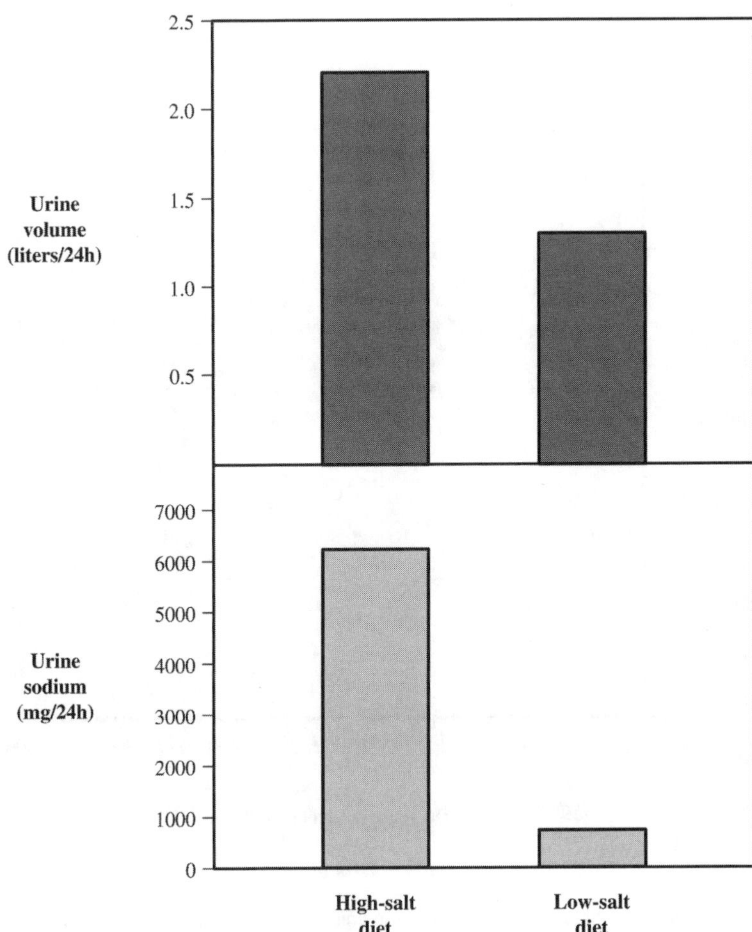

Fig. 1. Change in urine volume when volunteer subjects were switched from a high-salt to a low-salt diet (top). The difference was 0.9 liters in twenty-four hours. Change in urine sodium when subjects were switched from a high-salt to a low-salt diet (below). The difference was 5900 mg in twenty-four hours. (Reproduced with permission from He, FJ et al. Effect of salt intake on renal excretion of water in humans. *Hypertension* 2001;**38**:317–320)

tant factor in controlling urinary volume not only for hypertensive patients (in the He and MacGregor study) but also for normotensive persons (in the INTERSALT study).

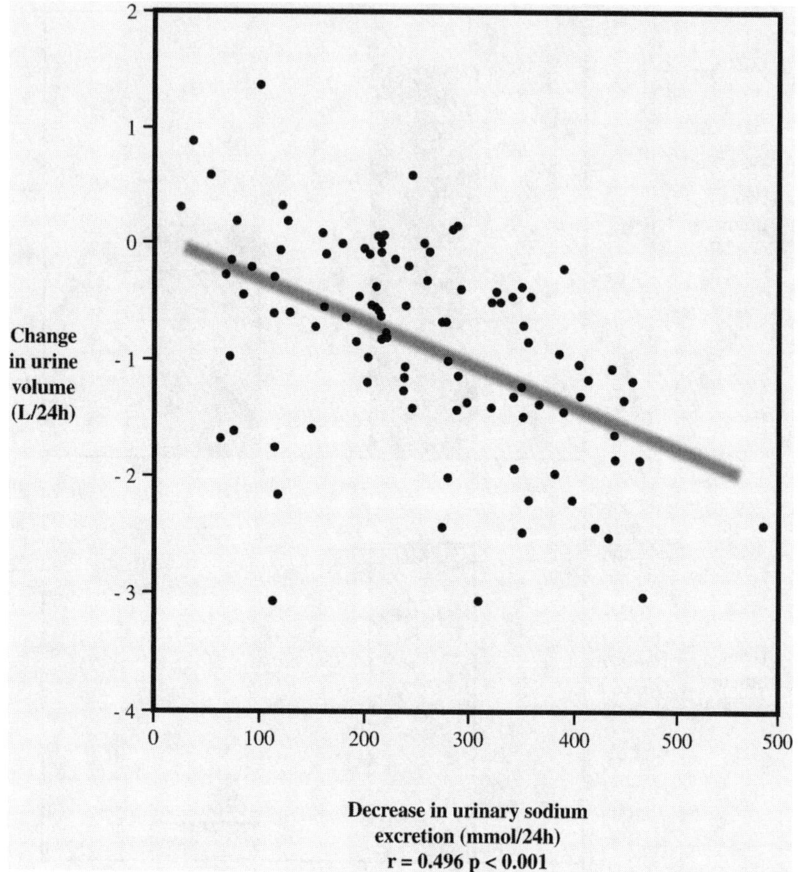

Fig. 2. Relationship between change in urine volume and change in urinary sodium excretion when subjects were switched from a high-salt to a low-salt diet. Shown: the intercepts for all 104 subjects and the calculated regression line. Urinary volume decreased by 160 ml for a 1000 mg reduction in sodium excretion. (Reproduced with permission from He, FJ et al. Effect of salt intake on renal excretion of water in humans. *Hypertension* 2001;**38**:317–320)

The results were not unexpected. Dietary sodium has long been known to stimulate thirst. Movie theaters position the soda fountain and the popcorn concession immediately adjacent to each other. Pubs make salty snacks readily available to their customers at little

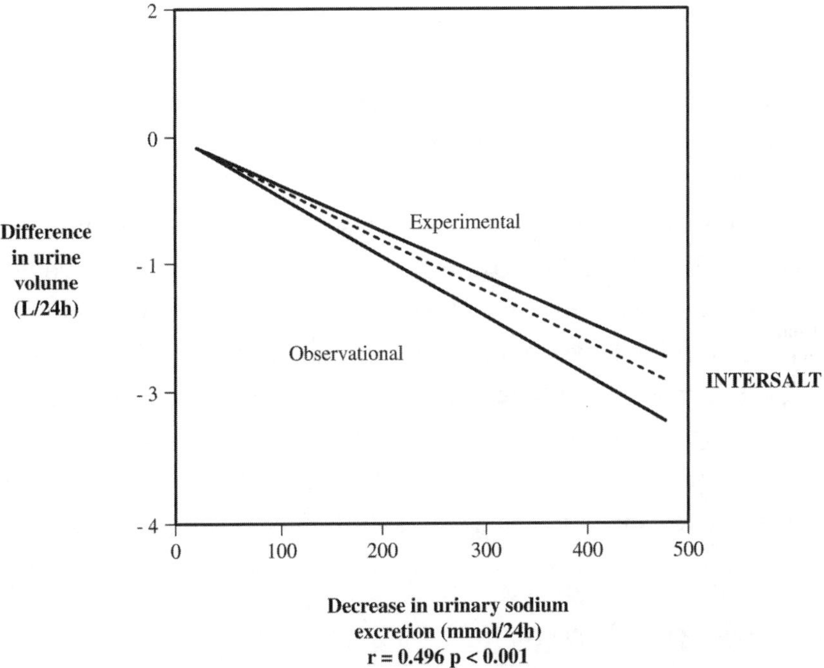

Fig. 3. Relationship between change in urine volume and change in urinary sodium excretion for the Experimental (104 subjects) and the Observational (637 subjects) studies of He, FJ et al. Also superimposed on the graph is the plot of INTERSALT data. The three studies show similar regression lines. The consistent results show that salt intake is an important factor controlling urinary volume. (Reproduced with permission from He, FJ et al. Effect of salt intake on renal excretion of water in humans. *Hypertension* 2001;**38**:317–320)

or no charge. Certainly, the Pepsi, Inc. executives were well aware, in 1962 when Pepsi and Frito-Lay merged into a colossal business enterprise, that the snacks of the latter would increase demand for Pepsi's beverages.

Since 1962, Frito-Lay has contributed mightily to the success of Pepsi's business.[5] Revenue for 2004, the latest available, comes in at $29 billion, some 600 times the 1962 amount.

Pepsi is not the only food manufacturer who understands the

symbiotic relationship between snacks with salt and beverages. Phillip Morris,[6] a snack and cigarette company, has $36 billion in cigarette sales per year and $20 billion in snack sales.[7] The company also has a controlling interest in Miller Brewing, which rings up $4 billion in annual sales.

Professors He and MacGregor estimate that a reduction in sodium intake from 3500 to 1150 mg, the DASH 2001 goal, would reduce fluid intake by 350 ml/day per person.[8] Approximately 25 percent of fluid intake in the United Kingdom is in the form of soft drinks, they note. The reduction in sodium intake would reduce the number of soft drink sales by 13 million per day, or 5 billion per year. In the United States, a 2000 mg reduction in sodium intake would reduce soft drink sales by 40 billion per year.

FAST-FOOD OUTLETS

Certainly, quick-service restaurants have taken advantage of the interdependency of sodium intake and thirst. The salinity of their menus, they no doubt realize, is a direct determinant of the number and size of the beverages they will sell.

Consider what is done to their most popular item, the hamburger. When a hamburger is purchased at a quick-service outlet, the sodium-containing seasoning agent that is applied to the patty during cooking and the condiments that are added to the patty after cooking increase the salinity by two or three times. The data of table 1 are illustrative: While the quarter-pound meat patty contributes only 200 mg to one's daily sodium intake, the completely garnished burger dispensed at most outlets is likely to contain 700 to 900 mg of sodium.

The fast-food patron is generally unaware of the salt that is added during the cooking process. The outlets, to be sure, do not make such

Table 1. Breakdown of Sodium Content for a Typical Fast-Food Hamburger

	mg sodium
Meat patty	200
Roll	200
Seasoning (salt)*	100
Ketchup	200
Mustard	50
Mayonnaise	50
Total	800

*applied to the meat patty

an admission in their advertising displays. Obviously, they would rather the public not know.

A patron can ask the waiter to hold the mayo or whatever. But a person is not inclined to request "hold the salt" if he is not aware that salt is routinely added during the cooking process.

The sodium content for hamburgers sold at the five leading quick-service outlets is shown in table 2. Comparative analysis is

Table 2. Fat and Sodium Content of Hamburgers and Cheeseburgers at Traditional Quick-Service Outlets[9]

	Calories	*Percent fat*	*Sodium (mg)*
McDonald's			
Hamburger	280	36	590
Quarter Pounder with cheese	530	38	1310
Big Mac	580	42	1090
Burger King			
Hamburger	310	39	580
Cheeseburger	360	44	790
Whopper	760	54	1000
Wendy's			
Classic Single	410	41	890
Big Bacon Classic	570	46	1460
Jack-in-the-Box			
Hamburger	250	32	610
Hamburger with cheese	300	40	840
Bacon Ultimate Cheeseburger	1120	61	2260
Whataburger			
Whataburger	607	44	1158
Whataburger w/bacon and cheese	809	50	2065

complicated by deluxe offerings such as cheeseburgers, double burgers, ultimate burgers, and the like. In any case, it is easy to conclude that the hamburgers dispensed by fast-food outlets contain excessive amounts of salt. Burger King, incidentally, is the only outlet that does not routinely apply a salt seasoning during cooking.

During the past few years the traditional fast-food restaurants have diversified their menu and offered entrée selections other than burgers, such as grilled chicken, fish, chili, baked potatoes, and the like. Those items also contain large amounts of salt (table 3). Some outlets now offer salads. The dressings, nevertheless, are consistently high in sodium (and fat).

A final consideration are the french fries that routinely come to the consumer heavily salted. Add another 390 mg of sodium for the fries.

SPECIALTY OUTLETS

In the 1960s, when fast-food restaurants began spreading across the United States, not all were hamburger outlets. Notable among the latter are Kentucky Fried Chicken and Pizza Hut. Their menus also tend to be very salty. KFC marinates all its chicken pieces in a seasoning that contains salt. It does not offer low-sodium pieces. At KFC there is no such thing as "you can have it your way."

Table 3. Fat and Sodium Content of Example Diversified Foods at Two Quick-Service Outlets[10]

	Calories	*Percent Fat*	*Sodium (mg)*
Jack-in-the-Box			
Chicken Supreme	710	50	1440
Wendy's			
Taco Supreme Salad	360	42	1090

Table 4. Fat and Sodium Content of Specialty Outlets[11]

	Calories	*Percent Fat*	*Sodium (mg)*
Kentucky Fried Chicken			
Breast—Extra Crispy	470	53	1230
Original Recipe Sandwich	450	44	940
Arby's			
Beef 'n Cheddar	480	46	1240
Roast Ham and Swiss	730	42	2180
Pizza Hut			
Personal Pan Pizza, cheese	630	40	1370
Spaghetti with Meat Sauce	600	20	910

Pizza has a high salt content because of the tomato paste, the cheese, and the toppings. A no-sodium tomato paste and a low-sodium cheese could be offered to the more discriminating customers, but no such marketing efforts have been made to date.

Table 4 shows the fat and salt content for three specialty outlets: Kentucky Fried Chicken, Arby's, and Pizza Hut.

NEWCOMERS

Newcomers that offer a variety of products appear on the scene from time to time. But the result is the same: high sodium content (table 5). All these companies realize that a reduction in sodium intake would cause the loss of hundreds of millions of dollars in sales of soft drinks.

Table 5. Newcomers—Fat and Sodium Content[12]

	Calories	*Percent Fat*	*Sodium (mg)*
Chick-Fil-A			
Chicken Sandwich	410	37	1300
Subway			
Cold Cut Trio—Classic	440	43	1680
Subway Club—7 Under 6	320	16	1300

BOTTLED WATER

Sales of bottled water in the United States have grown at a remarkable pace during the last few years. In 2001 the volume increased by more than 520 million gallons over 2000.[13] Per capita consumption grew to 19.5 gallons (table 6). Sylvia E. Swanson, president of the International Bottled Water Association, explained, "Our public education campaign to inform people about the importance of being properly hydrated has encouraged Americans to drink themselves to better health."[14] She does not acknowledge that the bottled water industry is a beneficiary of an excessive sodium content for the US diet. The appeal to the US populace is ingenious. The latter is encouraged to "drink water to maintain an athletic edge, sustain mental alertness, and flush-out impurities from the body."[15] A cynic might inquire of Swanson: Is sodium the impurity you are concerned about? Is it the impurity you want to flush out?

The perception that a copious amount of water is essential to good health is not founded in medical health. While it is true that the dietary excess of sodium must be carried out of the body in the urine, that function is not the implied intent of Swanson's recommendation.

For some, readily available portable water provides a sense of security (fig. 4). The fact that people are on the move as never before, from home to school to the workplace, makes it necessary

Table 6. US Bottled Water Market

Year	*Millions of Gallons*	*Annual % Change*	*Gallons Per Capita*
1991	2356	2.1	9.3
1992	2487	5.5	9.8
1993	2689	8.2	10.5
1994	2966	10.3	11.5
1995	3227	8.8	12.2
1996	3495	8.3	13.1
1997	3794	8.6	14.1
1998	4131	8.9	15.1
1999	4583	11.0	16.8
2000	4904	7.0	17.8
2001	5425	10.6	19.5

to relieve the sensation of thirst from a resealable, easy-to-carry bottle. A comparable sense of security could be provided by simply reducing dietary sodium so that thirst would be dampened to a more physiological level.

GATORADE

Gatorade, a sports drink, was developed/formulated in the late 1960s by the sports staff at the University of Florida.[16] Perspiration was collected from football players during practice sessions and subjected to laboratory analysis. Sodium was found, not surprisingly, to be the primary electrolyte constituent plus some potassium.

From those analyses Gatorade had its beginning. Originally, the beverage contained a large amount of sodium, but following criticism from the medical community, the soduim content was reduced. The amount the company settled on was 110 mg per eight-ounce container (table 7).

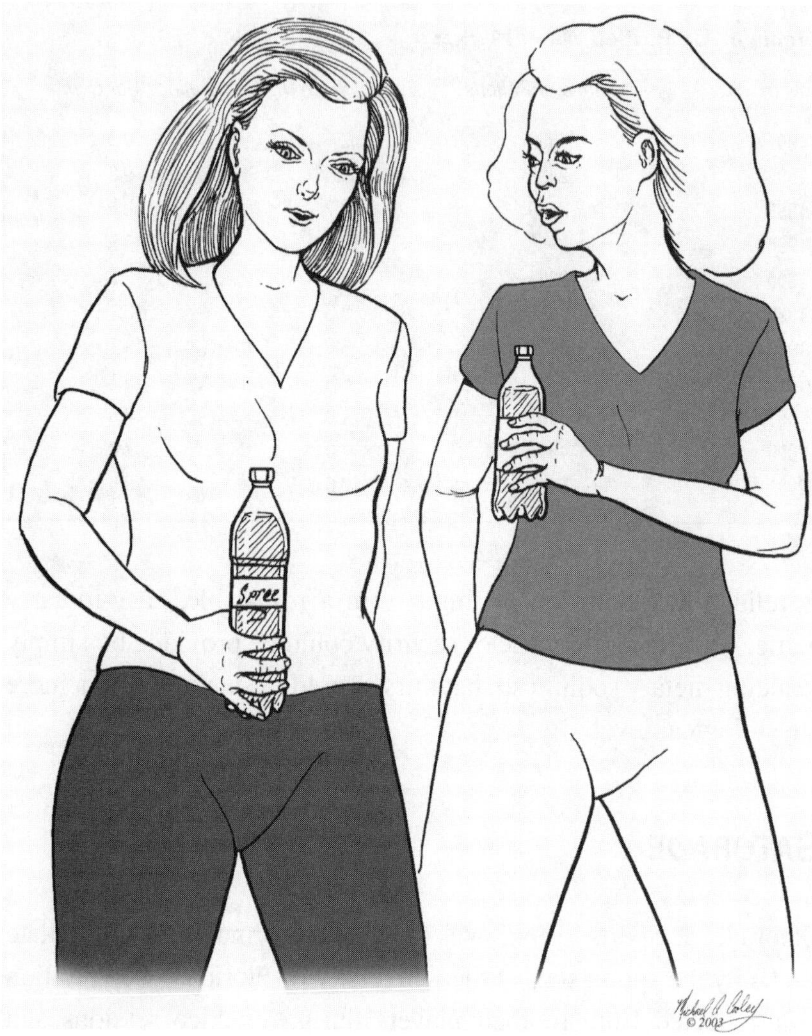

Fig. 4. Dietary salt stimulates thirst to such a degree that many find it necessary to carry with them a bottled beverage.

By 1984 sales of Gatorade totaled $100 million. In 2001 sales reached $2 billion worldwide.[17] Gatorade has experienced exponential growth with the sports and fitness craze that has swept through the United States during the past two decades. In 2001

Table 7. Electrolyte and Carbohydrate Content of Gatorade

	Sodium mg	*Potassium mg*	*Carbohydrate g*
Gatorade 8 oz.	110	30	14*

*equivalent to 50 calories

Gatorade and its subsidiary company Quaker Oats were purchased by Pepsi/Frito-Lay.

Gatorade bulletins have emphasized that only minor amounts of potassium, calcium, and magnesium are lost in sweat. Sodium, they note, is the primary constituent lost by far. And they conclude that the sodium should be replaced. But is it not reasonable to look at the other data? During a physically stressful situation, such as a midsummer preseason workout, the body attempts to rid itself, it seems reasonable to conclude, of an undesirable electrolyte. Most of the sodium lost in sweat could well be so explained. After all, the average US diet contains many times the minimal dietary requirement of sodium and low, if not insufficient, amounts of potassium, calcium, and magnesium. The low amount of potassium in perspiration might be the result of intentional conservation.

Gatorade executives are well aware that their products lack support from physicians. Their promotional activities avoid scrutiny within the medical/scientific arena and instead emphasize alliances with various professional and collegiate athletic programs. Gatorade promotes itself as the official sports drink of the National Football League, the National Basketball Association, the Women's National Basketball Association, the United Professional Golfer's Association, and Major League Baseball.[18] It also maintains exclusive relationships with numerous professional, collegiate, and amateur teams in the United States and throughout the world (fig. 5).

In addition to Gatorade Thirst Quencher, the corporation promotes other beverages with an array of electrolytic and nutrient components, such as Gatorade Energy Drink, which has a 20 percent carbohydrate component and *200 mg of sodium*; Gatorade Sports Nutrition Shake, which contains twenty-two vitamins along with protein (18 grams), electrolytes, and carbohydrates; and Propel, which has less sodium (35 mg per 8 oz.) than Gatorade. It also produces an energy bar and GatorLYTES, an electrolyte powder.[19]

SODIUM SUPPLEMENTATION IN A SPORTS BEVERAGE

What has been established by scientific research is that the sodium lost in perspiration is proportional to the amount consumed in the diet, just as sodium in the urine is a direct reflection of the dietary intake. The question arises, then: Should an athlete who adheres to a low-sodium fresh-food diet—a marathon runner from Kenya, for instance—replace fluid lost during strenuous activity with a sodium-fortified beverage such as Gatorade? Unfortunately, there are no studies that provide an answer. In fact, no studies have been done to indicate, at the other extreme, that an athlete who consumes excessive dietary sodium should replace fluid lost during exercise with a beverage such as Gatorade.

The Gatorade Web site material leads one to a different conclusion, though. The company states, in comparing the advantage of Gatorade to water: *Water lacks the electrolytes and energy that athletes need to perform at their best.* And for substantiation it lists one reference: Below, P.R. et al. *Med Sci Sports Exerc* 27: 200–210, 1995.

Retrieval of that study, which was performed at the University of Texas with the financial support of the Gatorade Sports Science Institute, reveals something different. Researchers within the Depart-

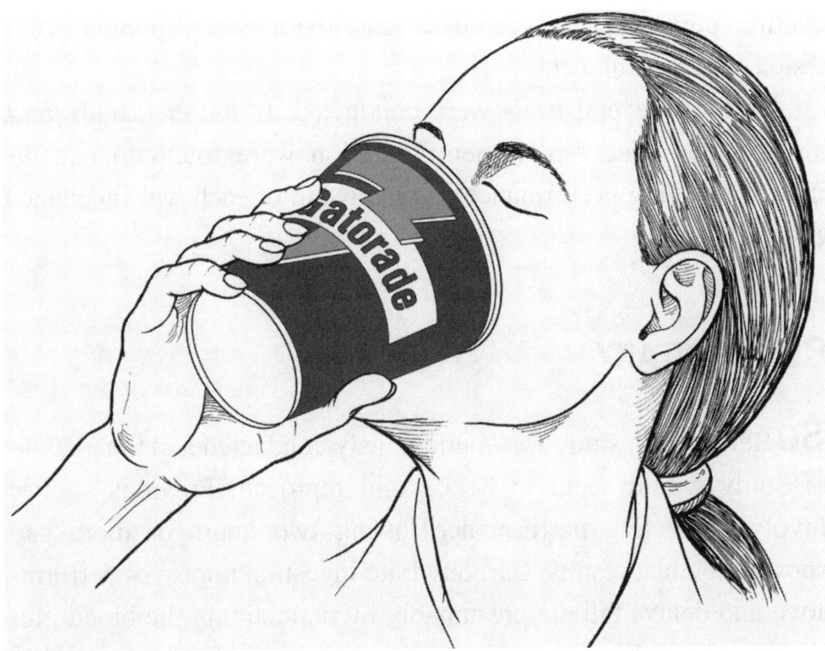

Fig. 5. Gatorade advertising is directed primarily toward children and young adults. The company sponsors little-league sports events and obtains preferential counter space during the contest. It pays professional sports franchises so that its products can be featured at athletic events. The company seeks exclusive rights with professional teams and uses that association to great advantage.[20]

ment of Kinesiology and Health Education tested the performance of cyclists during one hour of intense exercise. The subjects randomly received one of the following during the exercise bouts:

1. *Fluid and carbohydrate* in the form of Gatorade
2. *Fluid* in the form of a water-electrolyte solution
3. *Carbohydrate* in the form of a 40 percent maltodextrin-electrolyte solution
4. *Placebo* capsules containing electrolytes

Method. The participants were told that they would be receiving four different performance enhancers. During the trial, cycling performance as well as cardiovascular responses were tested for each subject.

Results. Several trials were conducted. In the end, both *fluid* and *carbohydrate* replacement ingestion were found to equally improve cycling performance and the result of each was independently additive.

COMMENTARY

The Below et al. study was meticulously conducted and the method of study would seem to be beyond reproach. Previous studies involving cycling performance lasting two hours or more had shown identical results. Carbohydrate ingestion improves performance and delays fatigue presumably by maintaining the blood glucose level and by preserving muscle glycogen.[21] Similarly, studies have shown that fluid replacement can delay fatigue.[22] The Below study, referenced by Gatorade in its Web site commentary, provided new findings in that performance was tested during a compressed, one-hour interval.

What was not tested was the perceived value, real or otherwise, of the electrolyte component. For each of the exercise bouts in the Below study, sodium was supplied, either by beverage or by capsule. There was no electrolyte differentiation among the four groups. Each group received sodium.

Water provides a competitive advantage and so do carbohydrates. But the jury is still out for electrolytes (sodium). Gatorade has no data to indicate that sodium in its beverage, either with or without potassium, enhances performance. In January 2003 that information was presented to the company by way of letter.[23]

The author's letter to the company read, in part:

> I noticed the following statement while reviewing your website information: **Water also lacks the electrolytes and energy that athletes need to perform at their best**. Included was the reference footnote: "Below, P.R. et al. *Med Sci Sports Exerc* 27:200–210, 1995."
>
> I then studied the Below et al. report and noted that their trial had nothing to do with electrolytes. You might turn to the experimental design portion of their report in which the authors state, "These experimental trials were chosen to fit a factional design to evaluate the main effects of the factors, fluid replacement and carbohydrate consumption, and the potential interaction between them."

Jeffrey J. Zachwieja, senior scientist for the Gatorade Sports Science Institute, in a letter dated March 13, 2002, replied as follows:

> You are right in that the study was not designed to specifically test for an electrolyte effect on exercise performance—in that sense the reference should have been attached to the energy portion of the statement instead of the entire statement. That said, I believe the Below research is still supportive of the general statement you have questioned. While the main experimental design focused on high volume vs. low volume fluid intake and carbohydrate vs. no carbohydrate intake . . . in essence, the study design can be viewed as systematically taking away active ingredients in Gatorade to test the effects on performance. Clearly all permutations were not tested, but the full complement (water, carbohydrate and electrolytes) did result in the best performance.

Well, the point is this: Gatorade (water, carbohydrate, and electrolytes) was not tested by Below et al. against a beverage containing only water and carbohydrate. Only such a trial will provide information regarding the value of the electrolyte component within

Gatorade. What must be maintained in such a study is participant blindness to the constituents that are being administered. That could be achieved, perhaps, by intravenous drip as the subject pedals a stationary bicycle. Surely, the sodium will prove, in a well-controlled scientific study, to be of no value at all. If so, that negative result should be released in a peer-reviewed scientific publication.

Gatorade has been on the market since 1972. Is it too much to ask of Gatorade executives: Why do you not have data, after thirty-plus years, to show, as you contend, that the sodium component in Gatorade enhances sports performance or, for that matter, is beneficial to one's general well-being? Furthermore, since no data exists, should you not forthrightly make that information known in your newsletters, your commercials, and your Web site material?[24] Finally, what information do you have regarding the daily sodium requirement for children involved in sports activities, to whom much of your sales promotion is directed, in comparison to that of adults performing similar activities?

It is all too apparent that Gatorade executives target children in their sales promotions, as did cigarette companies with their promotional campaigns fifty years ago. They know all too well that the electrolyte thirst quencher for the child becomes, in time, the addictive beverage for the adult.

MUSCLE CRAMPS

There is the perception among athletes and athletic trainers that the sodium component within a sports-enhancement beverage relieves the development of and, indeed, prevents the onset of muscle cramps. But testing of that hypothesis has not yet been rigorous. The experience of physicians has been confined primarily to the muscle cramps that patients with renal failure experience. Those cramps, in the lower extremities usually, occur toward the end of a hemodialysis session, when the blood pressure tends to fall and fluid balance has not been maintained.[25] Intravenous injection with dextrose and water immediately relieves dialysis cramps. Alternatively, sodium and water injection relieves the cramps. It has not yet been settled among nephrologists whether the decreased blood volume or a decrease of sodium in the bloodstream is responsible for the cramps. The fact that sugar with water relieves the cramps suggests that blood volume, that is, fluid depletion, is more important.

The causative factors responsible for the muscle cramps sustained by athletes have not been the subject of very much study. The only trials remotely relating to such cramps were performed in 1935 and 1936 by R. A. McCance.[26] His methods were not rigorous and both he and his subject's interpretation of the cramps are open to question.

Much needs to be done before athletes who sustain muscle cramps can be provided with advice that is well established by scientific data.

NOTES

1. Kanter, GS. Excretion and drinking after salt loading in dogs. *American Journal of Physiology* 1953;**174**:87–94.

Di Salvo, NA. Factors which alter drinking responses of dogs to intravenous injections of hypertonic sodium chloride solutions. *American Journal of Physiology* 1955;**180**:139–145.

Fitzsimons, JT. The effects of slow infusions of hypertonic solutions on drinking and drinking thresholds in rats. *Journal of Physiology* 1963;**167**:344–354.

2. Cowley, AW et al. Influence of daily sodium intake on vasopressin secretion and drinking in dogs. *American Journal of Physiology* 1983;**245**:R860–R872.

Eriksson, L and Valtonen, M and Makela, J. Water and electrolyte balance in male mink (*Nustela vison*) on varying dietary NaCl intake. *Acta Physiologica Scandinavica* 1984;**537(Suppl)**:59–64.

Denton, DA and Nelson, JF and Tarjan, E. Water and salt intake of wild rabbits (*Oryctolagus cuniculus* (*L*)) following dipsogenic stimuli. *Journal of Physiology* 1985;**362**:285–301.

3. He, FJ et al. Effect of salt intake on renal excretion of water in humans. *Hypertension* 2001;**38**:317–320.

4. The similar slope for the regression lines is a validation of sorts for the INTERSALT data. The Salt Institute had contested INTERSALT in 1996 on grounds that are inexplicable and continues to do so despite the confirmation supplied by He and MacGregor.

5. http://www.pepsi.com.

6. Philip Morris changed its name to Altria in April 2003.

7. http://www.philipmorris.com.

8. He, FJ et al. Effect of salt intake on renal excretion of water in humans. *Hypertension* 2001;**38**:317–320.

9. For further information refer to the Web site for a particular outlet.

10. Ibid.

11. For further information refer to the Web site for a particular outlet.

12. Ibid.

13. http://www.bottledwater.org.

14. http://www.bottledwater.org/public/pressrel. July 7, 1999.

15. Ibid.

16. http://www.gatorade.com.

17. Ibid.

18. The *Wall Street Journal* reported, on February 23, 2004, that Gatorade pays the National Football League $46 million a year in cash for right fees, which includes the privilege to station orange coolers and paper cups on the sidelines.

19. http://www.gatorade.com.

20. *Wall Street Journal*, February 23, 2004.

21. Coggan, AR and Coyle, EF. Carbohydrate ingestions during prolonged exercise: effects on metabolism and performance. In: *Exercise and Sport Sciences Reviews*, vol 19. Holloszy, JO (ed.). Philadelphia: Williams & Wilkins, 1991, pp. 1–40.

Coggan, AR and Coyle, EF. Effect of carbohydrate feedings during high-intensity exercise. *Journal of Applied Physiology* 1988;**65**: 1703–1709.

22. Barr, SI and Costil, DL and Fink, WJ. Fluid replacement during prolonged exercise: effects of water, saline, or no fluid. *Medicine & Science in Sports & Exercise* 1991;**23(7)**:811–817.

23. Research of the literature reveals no study that documents the need to replace sodium during sports events. Barr, SI (see note 22) assessed the need to replace sodium in endurance exercise ≤ 6 hours duration by comparing responses in fluid replacement with water, saline (25 mmol per liter), or no fluid. The subjects were cyclists. The authors concluded that their results clearly underscore the deleterious effects of dehydration. In contrast, the performance for subjects who received either water or saline was not significantly different. The authors concluded that the results indicate that sodium replacement does not appear to be necessary during events of moderate intensity and less than 6 hours duration; nevertheless, sodium loss was substantial.

24. It is also reasonable to ask of the Gatorade executives: Should children, whose cardiovascular and musculoskeletal system is not as fully developed as that of adults, be consuming the same sports beverage as that of adults?

25. McGee, S. Muscle cramps. *Archives of Internal Medicine* 1990; **150**:511–517.

26. McCance, RA. Experimental sodium chloride deficiency in man. *Proceedings of the Royal Society of London Biological Sciences* 1936; **119**:245–268.

McCance, RA. Sodium deficiencies in clinical medicine. *The Lancet* 1936;**1**:704–710, 765–768, 823–830.

CHAPTER 7

KIDNEY STONE (NEPHROLITHIASIS)

Go inside the nephrology clinic of a large metropolitan hospital and observe the planning of a much-needed, long-term clinical trial. At issue is the dietary recommendation that should be given patients who have experienced recurrent *kidney stone*, the term applied to the formation of calcium oxalate crystals within the pelvic portion of the kidney (fig. 1). The peak lifetime incidence for development of such a problem is in the fourth decade of life.[1] Males are affected more commonly than females.[2] Some 2 to 3 percent of the adult population develop kidney stone during their lifetime. As those afflicted will affirm, the striking feature of kidney stone is pain that starts in the posterior aspect of the flank, over the kidney, and often follows the course of the ureter (fig. 2), into the groin. That sensation recurs in spasmodic waves and increases with movement (migration) of the calcific particles from the pelvic portion of the kidney. Urinary urgency and frequency develop as the precipitates make their way down the ureter and into the bladder.

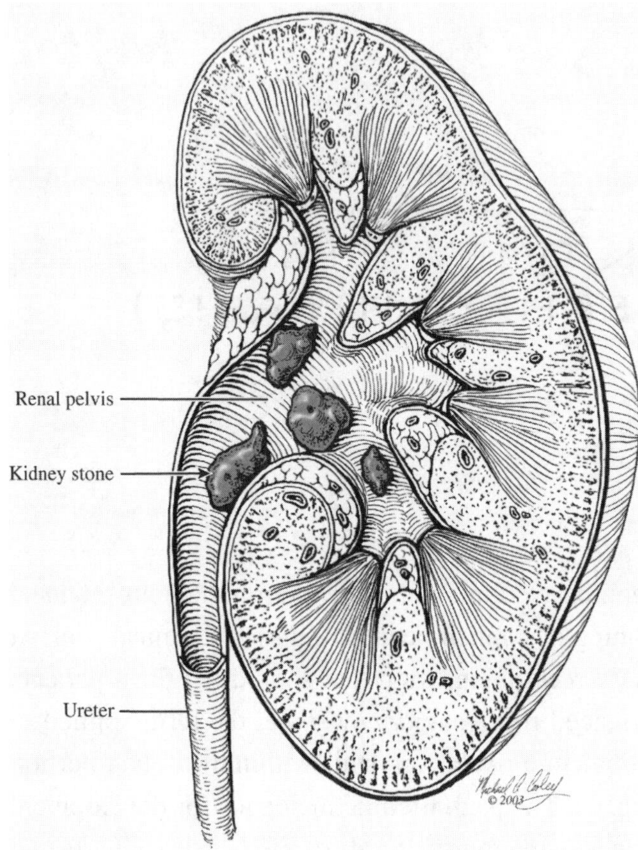

Fig. 1. Cross-sectional view of kidney, including pelvis and ureter. The funnel-shaped pelvis on the medial aspect of each kidney functions as the initial collection basin for the urine. It is in this area that calcium is capable of forming a stone. The ureter allows the urine to progress by the force of gravity to the bladder.

Kidney stone has a recurrence rate of 10 percent at one year, 35 percent at five years, and 50 percent at ten years.[3] What has long been sought by medical researchers is specific and effective dietary information that would lessen the likelihood of recurrence. In the past, a low-calcium diet has been the traditional advice. But recent studies[4] have shown that both dietary sodium and dietary protein play an important, if not preeminent, role in the development of kidney stone.

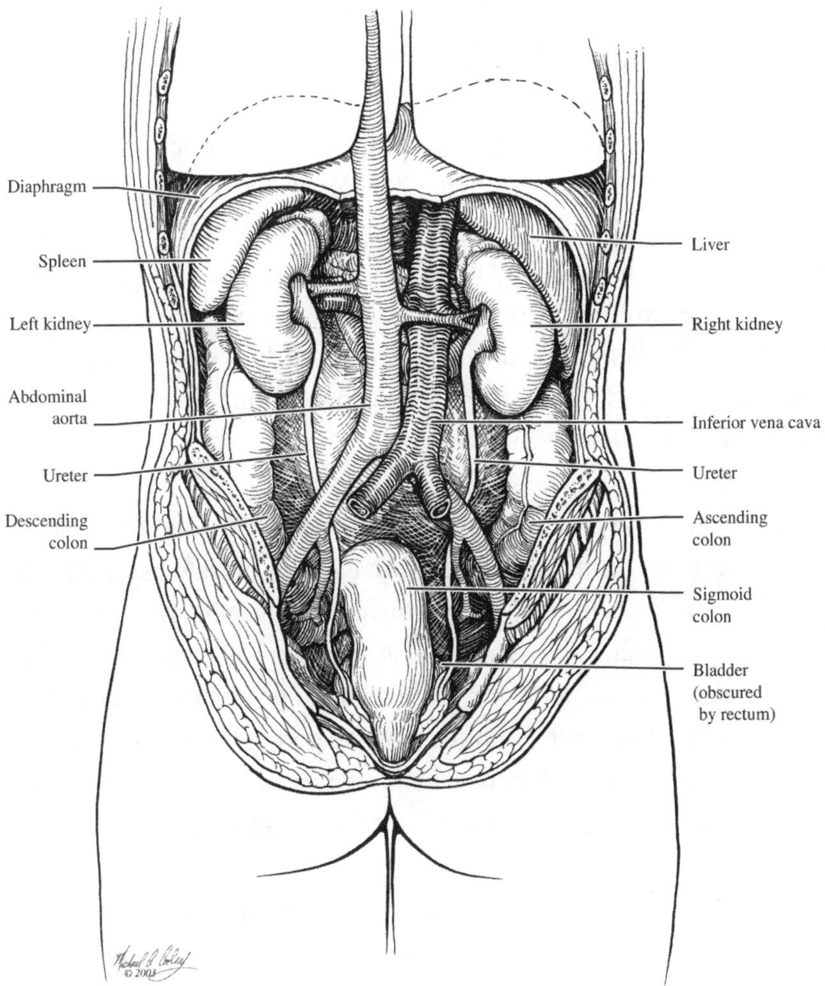

Fig. 2. Rear (dorsal) view of abdomen and lower body. From each kidney a tubular structure, the ureter, transmits urine to the bladder. The latter is situated immediately in front of the rectum and descending colon.

COMPARATIVE DIET STUDY FOR PREVENTION OF RECURRENT KIDNEY STONE

Confronted with unanswered questions, the Department of Clinical Sciences and Nephrology at the University of Parma in Parma, Italy, devised a clinical trial in the early 1990s that tested two contrasting dietary recommendations for kidney stone prevention. The results were published in a January 2002 issue of the *New England Journal of Medicine*.[5] In all, 120 patients, each of whom had previously experienced a calcium oxalate kidney stone (by far, the most common type), were involved.

A. Half of the group was assigned the traditional, often-prescribed regimen for those afflicted with calcium oxalate kidney stone: a low-calcium diet of 340 mg/day. Milk, yogurt, and cheese were specifically avoided. Water intake was increased to eight glasses a day to lessen the likelihood of particle precipitation (stone formation) within the pelvic portion of the kidney.

B. The remaining sixty patients were placed on a dietary regimen that was more complex and specific, containing (1) a generous amount of calcium, that is, 1000 mg per day, (2) a low amount of salt, that is, 1150 mg of sodium per day, with, finally, (3) a reduced protein intake of 52 g per day (in comparison to the normal intake of 70 g or so). Carbohydrates were increased with the additional consumption of vegetables, fruit, pasta, and the like. Water intake was increased to eight glasses a day, an instruction that was identical to that for the low-calcium group.

Randomization

The patients, all of whom were men, were asked to continue one or the other of the two dietary programs for at least five years.

Detailed information regarding all aspects of the study was carefully reviewed for each subject.

Results

The outcome measure was the time to which the first recurrence of a symptomatic kidney stone developed or the time to which the first indication of a stone could be identified by x-ray. A recurrence could be either symptomatic or silent.

Seventeen men did not complete the trial. At the five-year termination point, twenty-three of the sixty men on the low-calcium diet had recurrences while only twelve of the sixty men on the normal-calcium, low-sodium, and low-protein diet had recurrences. The cumulative incidence of recurrent stone development for the two groups is shown in figure 3. The risk of recurrence was found, on mathematical analysis, to be significantly less for the normal-calcium, low-sodium, low-protein group. The editorialist for the *New England Journal of Medicine*, David Bushinsky, MD,[6] noted that the Parma, Italy, results were groundbreaking and went on to say that a low-salt, reduced-protein, and ample-calcium diet would become, for medical physicians, the customary recommendation for the prevention of recurrent kidney stone.

The Relationship of Dietary Sodium and Dietary Protein with the Urinary Excretion of Calcium

Rarely does medical progress similar to that obtained by the Parma trial come out of nowhere. Medical researchers had long suspected that kidney stone was partly the result of excessive sodium and animal-type protein in the diet. Several studies over the past forty years had shown

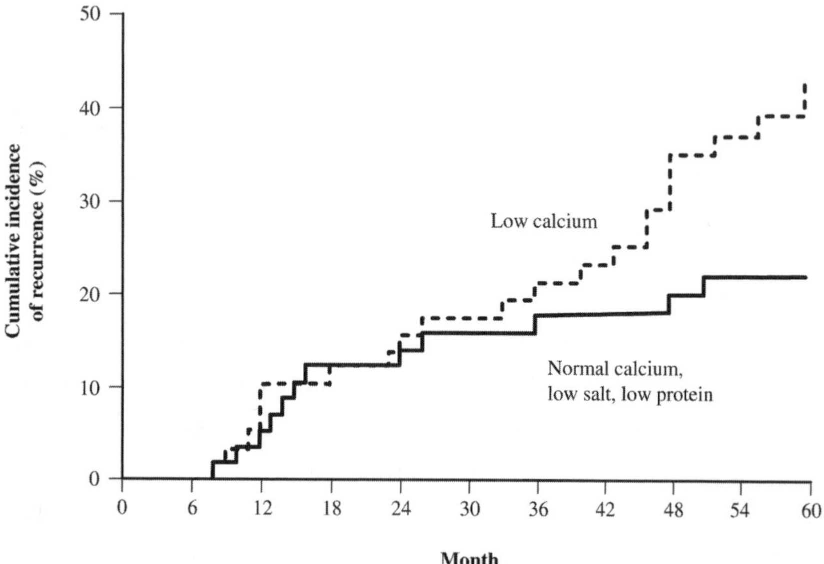

Fig. 3. Graphic demonstration of cumulative incidence for recurrent kidney stone according to assigned diet. The cumulative incidence for the subjects adhering to the normal-calcium, low-salt, low-protein diet was 22 percent. For the normal-diet, low-calcium group the cumulative incidence was 44 percent. Analysis showed that the relative risk of recurrence for the former group was statistically different from (less than) the risk for those in the latter group. (Reproduced by permission from Borghi, L et al. *New England Journal of Medicine* 2002;**346**:77–84, copyright 2002 Massachusetts Medical Society)

that *dietary sodium has a direct and powerful influence on urinary calcium excretion.*[7] Furthermore, *dietary protein* of the animal type *had been shown* in studies since 1979 *to also increase urinary calcium.*[8]

Dietary Sodium/Urinary Calcium

Modern work on the sodium/calcium relationship dates to M. Walser[9] whose classical experiments showed that a venous infusion of sodium raised urinary calcium in dogs. Subsequent trials have confirmed and broadened the concept of the sodium/calcium relationship. From the clinical point of view, the most notable single contributor to the medical literature has probably been A. Goulding, who demonstrated in a series of papers the dependence of urinary calcium on dietary sodium in both rats[10] and humans,[11] but others made important contributions, too.[12] The sodium/calcium effect takes place within the kidney, it is generally agreed, during the tubular reabsorptive phase. The initial filtration phase, which follows the perfusion of blood into the kidney, is unaffected by the dietary load of sodium.

It has long been realized that the kidney has three primary functions: (1) excretion of protein-catabolized wastes (urea, principally), (2) regulation of volume and compaction of body fluids (water and electrolyte excretion/secretion, acid-base control), and (3) regulation of blood pressure, distribution of blood flow (by hormonal activation/secretion). The kidney contains about one million functional units, each with a separate blood supply, filtration apparatus, and drainage (reabsorption) tubule. It is during transmission of urine through the tubule that sodium interferes with the reabsorption of calcium.

In recent years the dietary sodium load/urinary calcium excretion relationship has, for normal individuals, been represented quantitatively by researchers.[13] In a study involving normal male volunteers, an incremental increase of 1000 mg of dietary sodium causes the kidney to excrete (discard) 25 mg of calcium (fig. 4).[14]

One might think of the dietary sodium consumption/urinary calcium excretion relationship like this: The kidney is faced, daily, with the job of excreting the great excess of sodium that comes into the body as a result of dietary intake. Calcium becomes involved because calcium and sodium have a similar chemical structure. So, although calcium and sodium have markedly different roles to play in the body, calcium is not properly differentiated by the excretory apparatus in the kidney and, as a result, calcium is filtered into the urine along with the sodium.

M. Phillips and J. Cooke were the first to analyze, in 1967, the dietary sodium/urinary calcium relationship in subjects who had experienced kidney stone. They determined the twenty-four-hour urinary value for sodium and calcium under varying conditions of dietary intake.[15] For that group dietary sodium intake had a profound effect on urinary calcium excretion. Their data is presented in graphic form in figure 5. For every 1000 mg increase in sodium intake, the loss of calcium in the urine was 84 mg, or 3.4 times greater than the value found for normal subjects, as shown in figure 4. Calcium excretion for stone formers was found to be higher than that in normal subjects throughout all the experimental variations.

Silver et al. conducted similar experiments for stone-forming individuals. The dependence was only slightly less than that found by Phillips and Cooke, at 76 mg of calcium excretion for every 1000 mg of sodium.[16] Both Phillips and Cooke and Silver et al. sur-

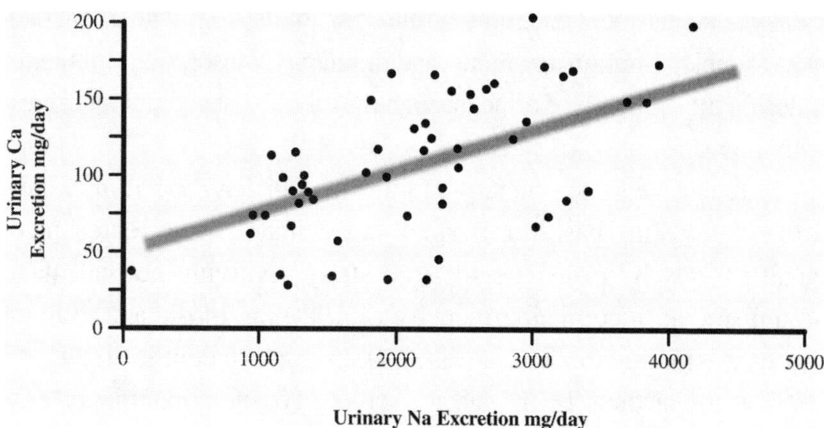

Fig. 4. Graphic correlation between the urinary excretion of sodium and calcium in normal male volunteers. The diet contained 400 mg of calcium per day for all individuals. Sodium intake was not limited. The slope of the line indicates that a 1000 mg change of sodium corresponds to 25 mg of calcium in normal individuals. (Modified from and reproduced with permission of Sabto, J et al. *Medical Journal of Australia* 1984;**140**:354–356) Note: urinary sodium excretion represents, almost identically, sodium consumption.

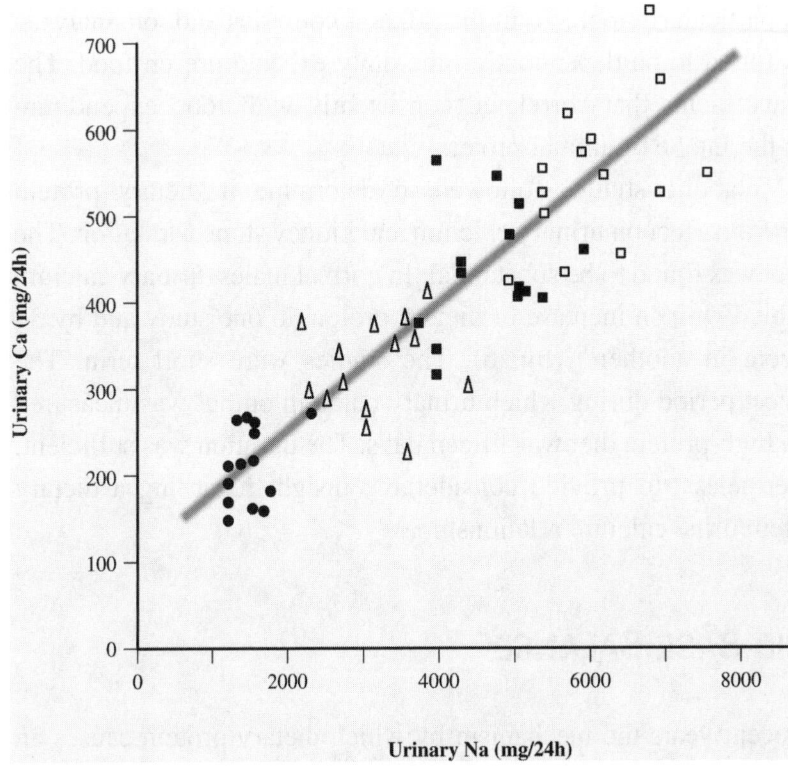

Fig. 5. Correlation between urinary sodium and calcium for stone-forming men. Four variations of sodium dietary regimens were employed. The slope of the curve, from data derived from four trials, indicates that a 1000 mg change in sodium corresponds to 84 mg of calcium. (Modified from and reproduced with permission of Phillips, MJ et al. *The Lancet* 1967;**1**:1354–1357, reprinted with permission from Elsevier) Urinary sodium corresponds to dietary consumption.

mised that sodium restriction should prove to be an effective method of preventing kidney stone formation.

Dietary Protein/Urinary Calcium

During the twentieth century the incidence of kidney stone gradually increased in the Western world.[17] The increased prevalence was particularly more so in the affluent countries and, on analysis, was found to be dependent on the daily expenditure on food. The dietary factor that correlated consistently with food expenditure was the intake of animal protein.[18]

Metabolic studies followed to determine if dietary protein exerts an effect on urinary calcium and kidney stone formation. The effect was found to be substantial. In normal males, urinary calcium doubled with an increase of dietary protein in one study and by 34 percent in another[19] (fig. 6). The studies were short term. The longest period during which urinary calcium output was measured on a high-protein diet was fifteen days. The duration was sufficient, nevertheless, to provide considerable insight regarding a dietary protein/urine calcium relationship.

ACID-BASE BALANCE

In recent years the mechanism by which dietary protein causes an increase in urinary calcium has been elucidated. Animal protein (from meat and cheese, for instance) contains sulfur-containing amino acids that are converted by the body's metabolic processes to sulfuric acid.[20] Vegetables and fruits, on the other hand, contain precursors of base in the form of organic anions (an electrolyte with a negative charge). The metabolic processes within the body are able to convert, with little effort, organic anions to bicarbonates (HCO_3).

Diets that are rich in animal foods and low in vegetable foods, typical of industrial countries, produce a net acid load that requires the alkaline effect of calcium for neutralization. Additionally, the types of protein present in the diet, because of their differing content of sulfur-containing amino acids, are final determinants of urinary net acid excretion and, in turn, calcium excretion. As shown in figure 7, when a group of healthy adults were fed a diet containing

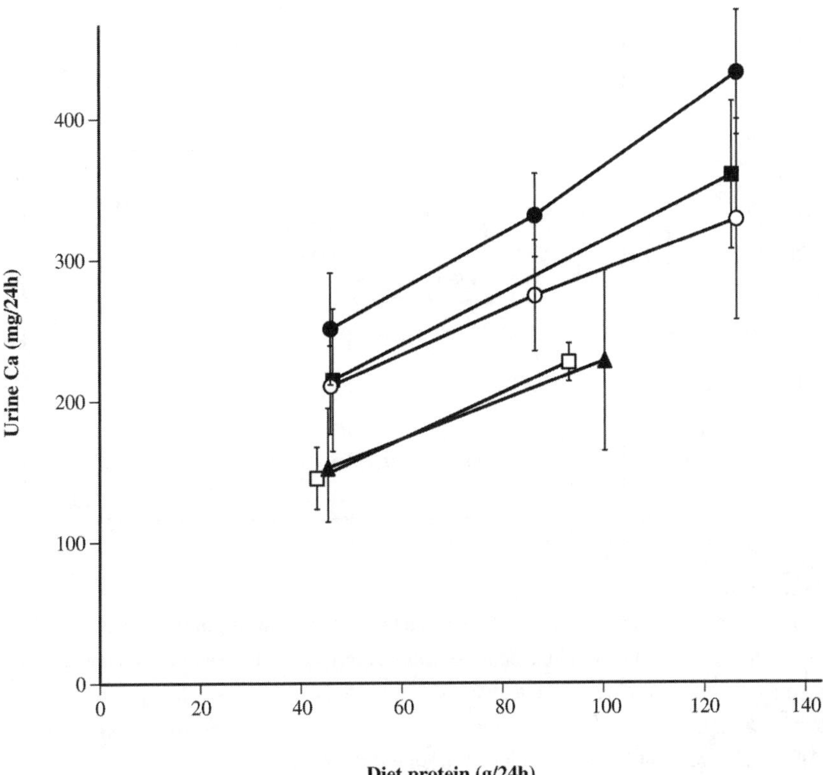

Fig. 6. Urinary excretion of calcium for subjects whose diet contained increasing amounts of protein. Urinary calcium rises progressively as protein intake increases (in otherwise constant diet). (Reproduced with permission from Lehman, J Jr. et al. *Kidney Int* 1996;**50**:341)

75 g of protein per day derived from vegetarian, ovo-vegetarian (vegetarian plus eggs), or animal protein sources while otherwise maintaining the composition of the diets constant, urinary net acid excretion and calcium rates rose progressively.[21]

Now, if one's diet contains an excess of animal protein, the buffering provided by fruits and vegetables might not be sufficient to maintain the desired level of acid-base balance. In that case, a

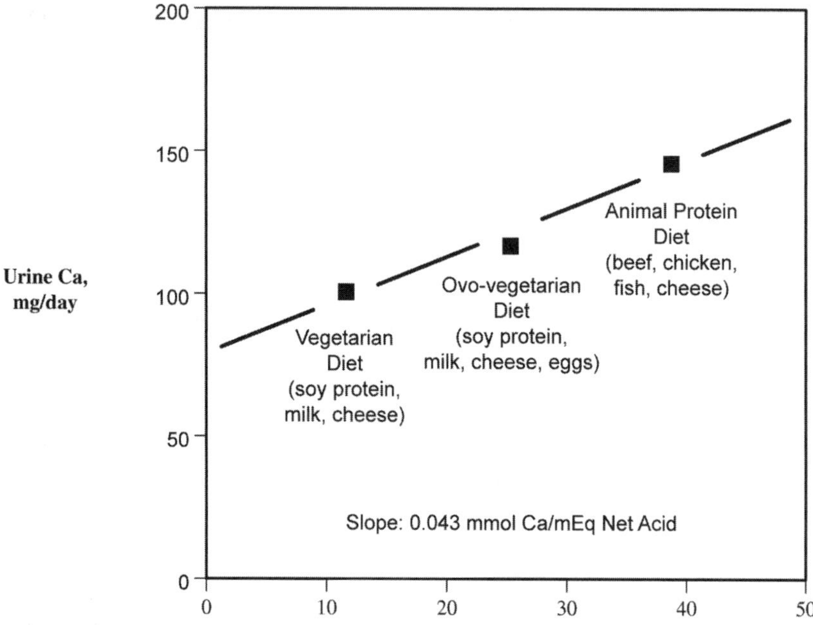

Fig. 7. When a group of healthy adults were fed 75 g protein/day derived from vegetarian, ovo-vegetarian, or animal sources while otherwise maintaining the composition of the diet constant, urinary net acid excretion and calcium excretion rates rose progressively. (Adapted from note 21 and reproduced with permission from Breslau, NA, et al. Relationship of animal protein–rich diet to kidney stone formation and calcium metabolism. *Journal of Clinical Endocrinology Metabolism* 1988;**64**:140–146)

secondary reservoir, skeletal bone, is mobilized to supply sufficient buffering of the sulfuric acid produced by animal protein.

Bone is well suited to an acid buffering role since it contains a large reservoir of alkaline salts that can be mobilized. The trade-off for protection of the acid-base equilibrium is the loss of mineral from bone. Biochemical analysis has shown that calcium is removed from bone in the form of an alkaline salt to neutralize the acids produced by proteins. Later, the calcium leached from bone is filtered into the urine by the kidney.

Kidney Function in the Twenty-First Century

For some time now scientists have realized that the kidney's function in today's modern man is very much different from that of yesterday's Stone Age man. The difference is the result of the alteration that has occurred in diet. The sodium intake for preagricultural man is estimated to have been 600 mg/day and the potassium level to have been 7000 mg/day. This is in stark contrast to recent data which estimate the daily intake of sodium and potassium at 4000 and 2500 mg respectively in the United Kingdom, the United States, and Australia. As noted by Eaton et al.,[22] the kidneys were designed to excrete more potassium than sodium because grains, nuts, fruits, vegetables, and meats were the staple of early man's diet. That evolutional mechanism still exists despite the reversal of sodium and potassium in the daily dietary consumption. The phrase "today's diet but yesterday's genes" is never more pertinent. What is surprising is that the flip-flop in dietary electrolytes which is, surely, largely responsible for kidney stone formation has not yet been recognized to be responsible for other kidney diseases, too.

Kidney Stone (Continued)

In the United States, kidney stone disease was responsible for an estimated 1.32 million visits to physicians in 1995 and for $1.83 billion in health costs in 1993. Once a kidney stone forms, there is a high probability that a second stone will develop. Appraisal of the factors responsible for stone formation in a long-term study became a top priority for the Parma University researchers. And, as a result of their efforts, over a several-year period, a low-salt, low-protein, ample-calcium, and abundant-water regimen was found to be significantly superior to the traditional low-calcium diet. As their recommendation is put into effect by nephrologists worldwide, now and in the future, a pronounced reduction in kidney stone disease can be expected to follow. The financial benefit resulting from decreased incidence in kidney stone will be appreciable.[23]

CALCIUM DEPOSITS IN ORGANS OTHER THAN THE KIDNEY

When calcium leaches from bones, as a result of dietary sodium excess, abnormal redeposition occurs in sites other than the kidney: for instance, gallstones contain calcium, in addition to cholesterol. Calcium can become deposited within the valves of the heart and restrict their function. Cholesterol plaques within the larger arteries of the body also attract calcium ions. And the ophthalmologist notices, on occasion, calcium deposition with the vitreous gel of the eye, so-called asteroid hyalitis (fig. 8).

SALT INSTITUTE

The medical reports regarding the kidney stone/dietary sodium relationship have not escaped the attention of the Salt Institute. And, predictably, the role of sodium in the causation of kidney stone was summarily dismissed. In remarks to the World Health Organization, Salt Institute president Richard L. Hanneman[24] remarked, without scientific substantiation: "No expert in stone disease would argue for restricting salt [for the prevention of kidney stone]; he or she would recommend water and mineral repletion."

Whoa. For the prevention of stone formation, the dietary recommendation of the Parma study and the *NEJM* editorial staff was (a) unrestricted dietary calcium and (b) a low-salt and low-protein

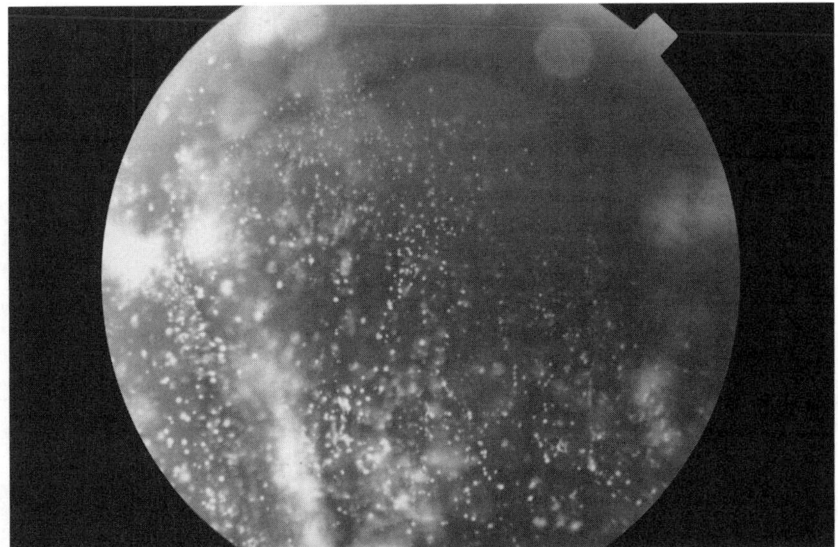

Fig. 8. Left eye, calcium deposits within vitreous gel (asteroid hyalitis).

dietary regimen. No one would disagree with the Salt Institute's recommendation of water repletion, but mineral repletion requires further explanation. The Parma investigators showed that less, not more, sodium is necessary in order to prevent recurrent stone formation. Before Hanneman of the Salt Institute comments further regarding this subject, he will, hopefully, consult with medical researchers who are knowledgeable of the effect that dietary sodium exerts on urinary calcium excretion.

Diet and Calcium

Advocates of high-fat and high-protein diets—Colker (*The Greenwich Diet*), Atkins,[25] Somers, Eades (*Protein Power*), Herman Tarnower (*The Complete Scarsdale Medical Diet*)—pay no respect to the ramifications of calcium metabolism in the books they have authored. Indeed, nowhere in their books is there an admission that dietary excess of sodium pulls calcium into the urine or that a high-protein diet causes calcium leaching from bone for maintenance of acid-base balance. Osteoporosis and kidney stone formation are two health issues that are conspicuous as a result of their absence in the writings of the high-fat high-protein proponents.

NOTES

1. Pak, CYC. Citrate and renal calculi. *Mineral and Electrolyte Metabolism* 1987;**13**:257–266.

2. Sutherland, JW et al. Recurrence after a single renal stone in a community practice. *Mineral and Electrolyte Metabolism* 1985;**11**: 267–269.

3. Ibid.

4. Silver, J et al. Sodium dependent idiopathic hypercalciuria in renal-stone formers. *The Lancet* 1983;**2**:484–486.

Lemann, J Jr. Relationship between urinary calcium and net acid excretion as determined by dietary protein and potassium: A review. *Nephron* 1999;**81(Suppl** 1):18–25.

5. Borghi, L et al. Comparison of two diets for the prevention of recurrent stones in idiopathic hypercalciuria. *New England Journal of Medicine* 2002;**346**:77–84.

6. Bushinsky, DA. Recurrent hypercalciuric nephrolithiasis—does diet help? Editorial. *New England Journal of Medicine* 2002;**346**:124–125.

7. Kleeman, CR et al. Effect of variations in sodium intake on calcium excretion in normal humans. *Proceedings of the Society for Experimental Biology and Medicine* 1964;**115**:29–32.

Phillips, MJ and Cooke, JNC. Relation between urinary calcium and sodium in patients with idiopathic hypercalciuria. *The Lancet* 1967;**1**: 1354–1357.

Breslau, NA et al. The role of dietary sodium on renal excretion and intestinal absorption of calcium and on vitamin D metabolism. *Journal of Clinical Endocrinology and Metabolism* 1982;**55**:369–373.

Muldowney, FP and Freaney, R and Moloney, MF. Importance of dietary sodium in the hypercalciuria syndrome. *Kidney International* 1982;**22**:292–296.

8. Robertson, WG et al. The effect of high animal protein intake on the risk of calcium stone formation in the urinary tract. *Clinical Science* (Colch) 1979;**57**:285–289.

Allen, LH and Oddoye, EA and Margen, S. Protein-induced hypercalciuria: a longer term study. *American Journal of Clinical Nutrition* 1979; **32**:741–749.

Zemel, MB et al. Role of the sulfur-containing amino acids in protein-induced hypercalciuria in men. *Journal of Nutrition* 1981;**111**:545–552.

Lemann, J Jr. et al. The importance of renal net acid excretion as a determinant of fasting urinary calcium excretion. *Kidney International* 1986;**29**:743–746.

9. Walser, M. Calcium clearance as a function of sodium clearance in the dog. *American Journal of Physiology* 1961;**200**:1099–1104.

10. Goulding, A. Effects of dietary NaCl supplements on parathyroid function, bone turnover and bone composition in rats taking restricted amounts of calcium. *Mineral and Electrolyte Metabolism* 1980;**4**:203–208.

11. Goulding, A. Fasting urinary sodium/creatinine in relation to calcium/creatinine and hydroxyproline/creatinine in a general population of women. *New Zealand Medical Journal* 1981;**93**:294–297.

Goulding, A. Effects of dietary salt intake on the fasting urinary excretion of sodium, calcium and hydroxyproline in young women. *New Zealand Medical Journal* 1983;**95**:850–854.

12. Kleeman, CR et al. Effect of variations on sodium intake on calcium excretion in normal humans. *Proceedings of the Society for Experimental Biology and Medicine* 1964;**115**:29–32.

Breslau, NA et al. The role of dietary sodium on renal excretion and intestinal absorption of calcium and on vitamin D metabolism. *Journal of Clinical Endocrinology and Metabolism* 1982;**55**:369–373.

Bringhurst, FR and Potts, JT. Calcium and phosphate distribution, turnover and metabolic actions In: *Endocrinology*. DeGroot, W et al. (eds.). New York: Grune and Stratton, 1999;**2**:551–585.

13. Nordon, BE. The nature and significance of the relationship between urinary sodium and urinary calcium in women. *Journal of Nutrition* 1993;**123**:1615–1622.

14. Sabto, J et al. Influence of urinary sodium on calcium excretion in normal individuals. *Medical Journal of Australia* 1984;**140**:354–356.

15. Phillips, MJ and Cooke, JNC. Relation between urinary calcium and sodium in patients with idiopathic hypercalciuria. *The Lancet* 1967;**1**:1354–1357.

16. Silver, J. Sodium-dependent idiopathic hypercalciuria in renal-stone formers. *The Lancet* 1983;**2**:484–486.

17. Anderson, DA. Environmental factors in the aetiology of urolithiasis. In: *Urinary Calculi*. Cifuentes Delatte, L and Rapado, A and Hodgkinson, A and Karger, B. (eds.). 1973, pp. 130–144.

Sierakowski, R et al. The frequency of urolithiasis in hospital discharge diagnoses in the United States. *Investigative Urology* 1978;**15**:438–441.

18. Robertson, WG et al. *The risk of calcium stone formation in relation to affluence and dietary animal protein*. In: *Urinary Calculus*. Brockis, JG and Finlayson, B (eds.). Littleton, MA: PSG Publishing Company, 1979, pp. 3–12.

19. Lutz, J. Calcium balance and acid base status of women as affected by increased protein intake and by sodium bicarbonate ingestion. *American Journal of Clinical Nutrition* 1984;**39**:281–284.

Johnson, NE and Alcantara, EN and Linkswiler, H. Effect of level of protein intake on urinary and fecal calcium and calcium retention of young adult males. *Journal of Nutrition* 1970;**100**:1425–1430.

Schuette, SA and Zemel, MB and Linkswiler, H. Studies of the mechanism of protein-induced hypercalciuria in older men and women. *Journal of Nutrition* 1980;**110**:305–331.

20. Kleinman, JG and Lemann, J Jr. *Acid production*. In: *Clinical Disorders of Fluid and Electrolyte Metabolism*. 5th ed. Narins, RG (ed.). New York: McGraw-Hill, 1993, pp. 187–202.

Sebastian, A et al. Improved mineral balance and skeletal metabolism in post-menopausal women treated with potassium bicarbonate. *New England Journal of Medicine* 1994;**330**:1776–1781.

21. Breslau, NA et al. Relationship of animal protein-rich diet to kidney stone formation and calcium metabolism. *Journal of Clinical Endocrinology and Metabolism* 1988;**66**:140–146.

22. Eaton, SB. An evolutionary perspective enhances understanding of human nutritional requirements. *Journal of Nutrition* 1996;**126**:1732–1740.

23. Parks, JH and Coe, FL. The financial effect of kidney stone prevention. *Kidney International* 1996;**50**:1706–1712.

24. http://www.saltinstitute.org/pubstat/fnb.html.

25. Robert Atkins and Herman Tarnower died in 2003 and 1980, respectively.

CHAPTER 8

OSTEOPOROSIS

Osteoporosis, a resorptive (dissolution) process involving bone tissue, is a major health concern for people who live beyond the age of thirty-five. Bones have a dense outer surface like ivory and a spongelike interior. In the osteoporotic process the holes enlarge and bone mass (weight) decreases. Skeletal strength decreases and the susceptibility to fracture increases.

The resistance to the resorptive process varies. The cortical bones of the arms and legs have a compact microarchitecture that makes them more resistant to dissolution. On the other hand, low-density bones like vertebrae, which are designed for flexibility, are spongy and less resistant to the osteoporotic process.

THE VERTEBRAE

The vertebral column is made up of thirty-three vertebrae, arranged as follows: seven cervical, twelve thoracic, five lumbar, five sacral, and four coccygeal. The two latter groups are fused to form composite bones, the sacrum and os coccgis.

The weight-bearing body (pedestal portion) of a vertebra is particularly susceptible to the development of osteoporosis. The resorption produces vertical compression within the vertebral body over time that, in the advanced stage, can progress to fracture and collapse (fig. 1).

In the upper back the thoracic vertebrae are prone to anterior compression and the assumption of a wedge-shaped configuration. As a result, the spine tilts forward and an individual so afflicted becomes humpbacked and stooped shouldered (fig. 2). The medical term for anterior compression of the spine is *kyphosis*. The lay description is dowager's hump. Women, whose bone mass is less, are more susceptible to osteoporotic deterioration of vertebrae than men.

An early indication of kyphosis is loss of height. Usually, the spinal deformation resulting from the anterior angulation does not cause pain, but loss of balance and difficulty in walking can be bothersome, with progression of the kyphotic affliction. In the lower back, or lumbar region, osteoporosis causes compression of the entire vertebral body. Height becomes diminished (fig. 2). Unlike the development of kyphosis within the upper back, pain within the lower lumbar region is often bothersome, yet nerve impingement is infrequent.

Osteoporosis involving the hip and the major leg bone (the femur) gives rise to fracture from falls of relatively minor severity (fig. 3). Low serum vitamin D levels are often found in such patients.[1]

Loss of balance and impaired agility contribute to the occurrence of such events. Hip fracture is frequent in the elderly, and even with successful execution of the corrective surgical procedure,

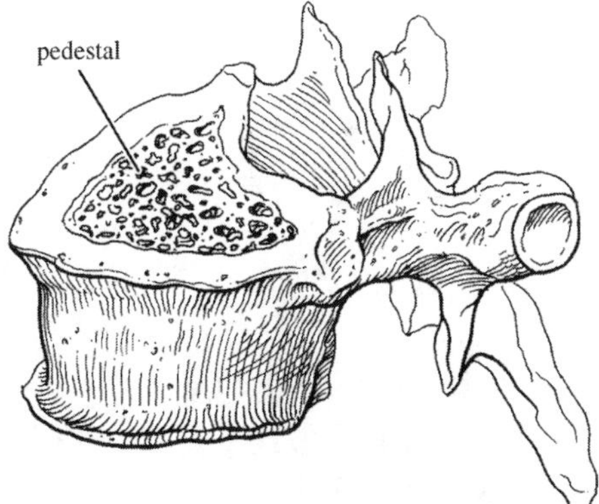

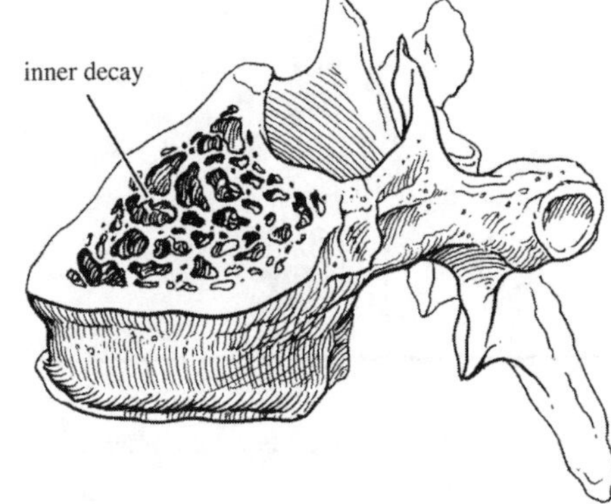

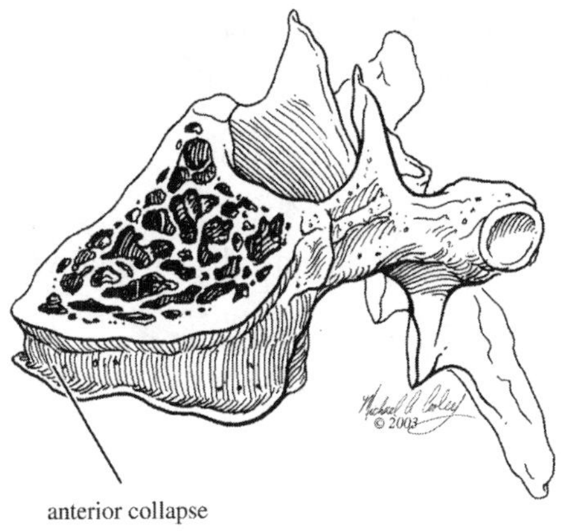

Fig. 1. Progression of osteoporotic decay for the upper, or thoracic, vertebrae. The pedestal, or weight-bearing portion of a vertebra, is prone to sustain anterior, or wedge-shaped, collapse. The result: an anterior tilt to the spinal column. Note increasing porosity.

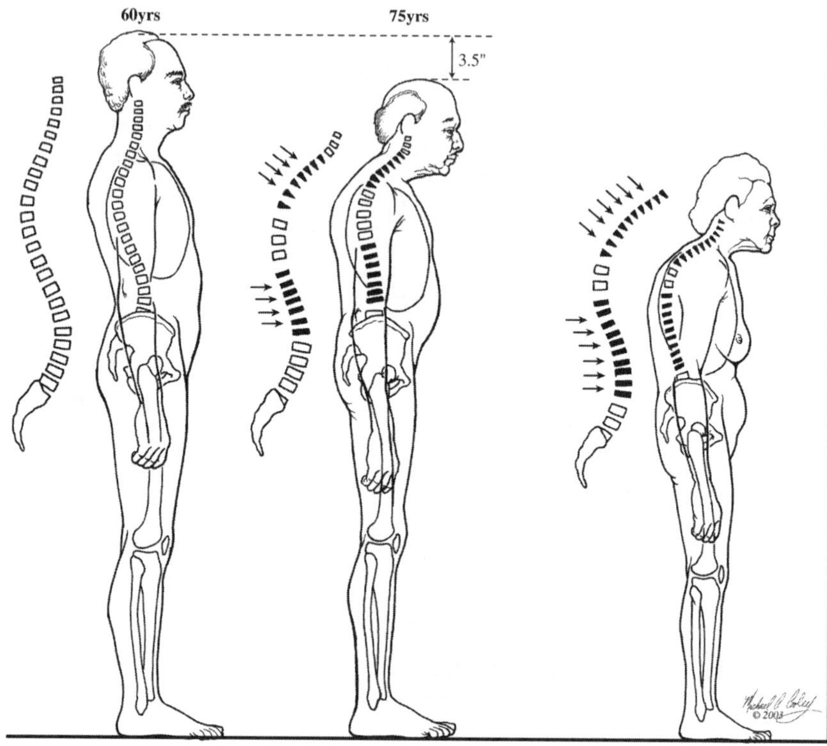

Fig. 2. Diagrammatic representation of osteoporotic decay for the spinal column. Wedge-shaped collapse of vertebrae in the upper thoracic column causes dowager's hump, or kyphosis, with a 1 1/2 to 2" loss of height. Compression of vertebrae within the lower back can cause an additional 1 1/2 to 2" loss of height. Note loss of waistline and protuberant abdomen. The vertebral collapse within the lower back often produces nerve impingement and chronic pain.

healing can be a slow process. Permanent impairment of ambulation and in the performance of routine tasks such as getting out of bed can be the late result of such fractures.

Impaired ambulation accelerates the osteoporotic process and makes one susceptible to additional fractures.

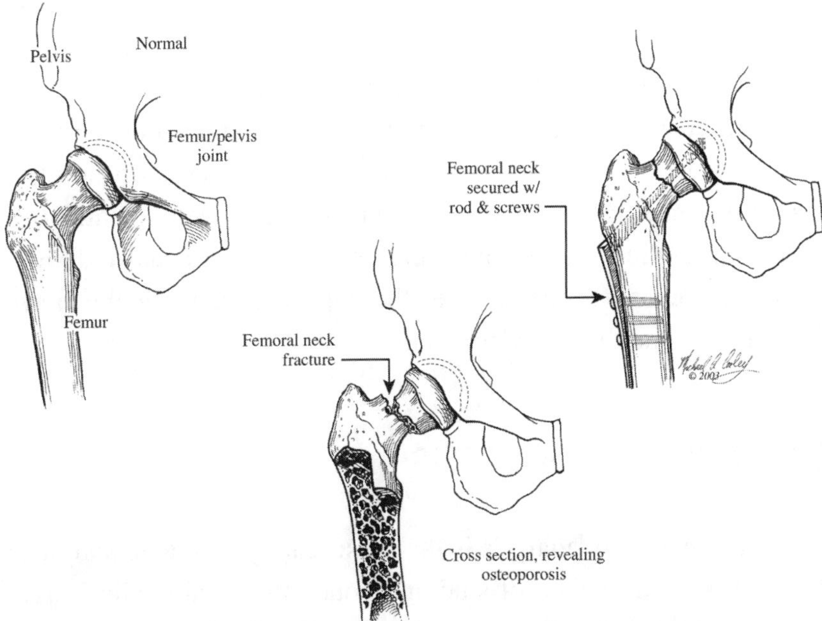

Fig. 3. Femur-pelvis articulation (hip joint). **Left:** Normal skeletal anatomy. **Middle:** Fracture of femoral neck. **Right:** Surgical repair.

THE SKELETON

The function of bone is to provide support, protection, and critical electrolytes for cellular activity. The mineral component of bone is a calcium and phosphorus matrix in the form of hydroxyapatite $[Ca_{10}(Po_4)6(OH)_2]$.

The lifetime cycle for body bone mass is shown diagrammatically in figure 4. Peak bone development occurs at age 25–30, which is about ten years following cessation of linear growth.[2] After a five- to ten-year plateau, total bone mass begins to decline. For women, in midlife especially, the decline proceeds at a faster rate than for men, sometimes approaching a 1.0 percent loss of bone mass per year. Often, at age eighty the bone mass for a woman is an astonishing one-half the earlier maximum! The decline for men is 33 to 50 percent less than that for women.[3]

Bone mass is dependent on body size. Peak bone development is less for women than it is for men primarily because of the body size difference. Ethnicity also influences bone development. Bone density is less in white people than in African Americans[4] and Mexican Americans.[5] Asian people, the Japanese in particular, have less-dense bone than do Caucasians.[6]

DEFINING OSTEOPOROSIS

Conventional x-ray analysis is the most readily available and most frequently used method of studying bone in clinical medical prac-

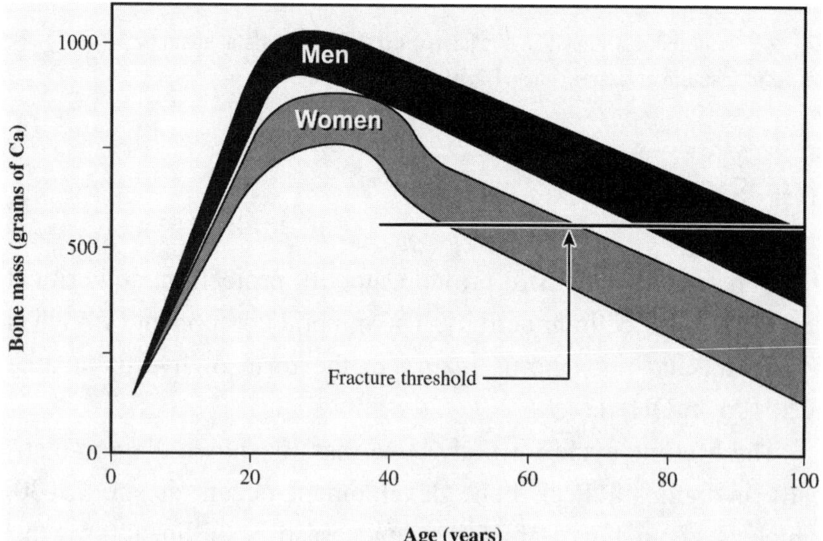

Fig. 4. Graphic representation of total skeletal weight in grams, birth to old age. Peak bone mass develops at age thirty and decays in later adult life. Fracture threshold is estimated. The difference between young men and women shown in this figure is largely a matter of body size. (Reproduced with permission from *Osteoporosis: Diagnosis and Management*, by G. R. Mundy. Martin Dunitz, Ltd., publisher)

Table 1. World Health Organization Classification of Low Bone Mass
Normal: Bone mass density (BMD) not more than 1 standard deviation below the young adult mean.[7]
Osteopenic: BMD between 1 and 2.5 standard deviations below the young adult mean.[8]
Osteoporosis: BMD more than 2.5 standard deviations below the young adult mean.
Established (or severe) osteoporosis: BMD more than 2.5 standard deviations below the young adult mean in the presence of one or more fractures.

tice. X-rays provide detailed visualization of bone and give some information as to its structure. The progressive collapse of vertebrae or the commencement of a fracture in a long bone can be gauged. Also, the thickness of the outer layer, the *cortex*, and the density of the inner framework, the *trabeculum*, can be analyzed.

X-rays do not allow for the determination of bone mineral content at deep sites when there is much surrounding soft tissue. For that analysis a radioisotope was perfected, employing a process known as *dual photon absorptiometry*. The radioisotope source is beamed through the bone, in a limb for instance, and the radiation that passes through is recorded by a collimated scintillation counter. The bone mineral content per unit area is calculated from the photon absorption following standardization. For deep sites, such as the femoral neck or the lumbar vertebrae, two different photon energies are necessary. The method, dual photon absorptiometry, has high precision and accuracy.

In 1987 dual x-ray absorptiometry replaced the radioactive source with an x-ray tube. Scan times were reduced to six minutes. Resolution and precision were substantially improved.

As bone density decreases, in the osteoporotic process, some bones resorb faster than others. Because the gradient of increasing

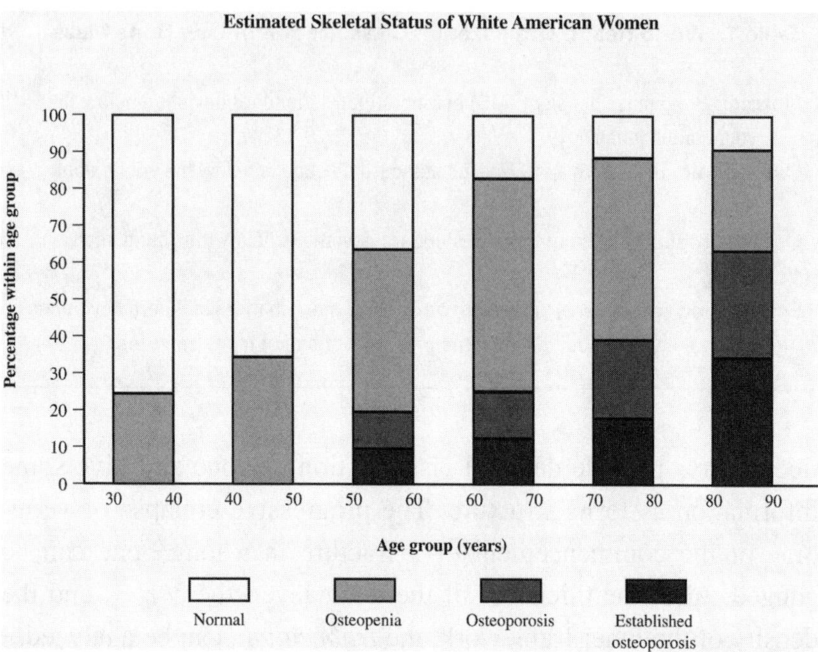

Fig. 5. Estimated skeletal status of white American women by age decade using WHO criteria. (Reproduced with permission from *Osteoporosis: Diagnosis and Management*, by G. R. Mundy. Martin Dunitz, Ltd., publisher)

fracture risk is imprecise, it is necessary to arbitrarily assign clinical significance to a level of bone loss. Bone density measurements provide the accurate and reproducible means of determining bone mass and of assigning clinical significance. That result is compared to the bone mass measurement for a normal thirty-year-old. Osteoporosis is defined on the basis of standard deviation from the norm[9] (table 1).

THE SIZE OF THE PROBLEM

Clinical studies have confirmed that most American women under the age of fifty have a normal bone mineral density. With advancing age, an increasing number have decreased bone density, so that by age eighty, 21 percent are osteopenic (moderate loss) and 70 percent have osteoporosis (marked loss)![10] (See fig. 5.) Sixty percent of the latter group will have experienced one or more fractures by age eighty. It is estimated that in the United States 16.8 million women are osteopenic and a further 9.4 million are osteoporotic.[11]

For the population at large, the lifetime risk of developing a fracture as a result of osteoporosis is 39.7 percent for women and 13.1 percent for men.[12] Women experience fractures earlier, but by age eighty the age-specific incidence for men approaches that for women.

Is Osteoporosis a Disease?

The notion that 45 percent of women age fifty and over have osteopenia (moderate loss of bone) raises philosophical questions about whether a condition so common should be considered a disease or part of the "normal" aging process. In the final analysis, the issue is philosophical only in argumentative terms since osteopenia leads to fractures and fractures lead to substantial adverse health outcomes. For example, in a Rochester, Minnesota, study[13] among women age eighty years and over who had osteopenia, 47 percent had already experienced one or more fractures, but the comparable figure among the oldest women without osteopenia was only 25 percent. Since it has been demonstrated that low bone mass is a major risk factor for fractures and is, moreover, preventable, it has seemed reasonable to some researchers to include osteopenia within the scope of osteoporosis. If a condition causes huge health-care costs and can be favorably affected by intervention and treatment, then it can only be considered to be a disease.

Both osteopenia and osteoporosis have been shown on the basis of decreased bone mineral measurements to be a very common problem. The size of the population affected by osteoporosis is not without precedent, however, in comparison to some other chronic diseases. For example, 36 percent of the age fifty and over women in Rochester, Minnesota, where the incidence of osteopenia and osteoporosis has been meticulously documented, also had hypertension.[14]

Over their lifetime a majority of white women, the most susceptible group by gender and ethnicity, are affected by osteoporosis, as are many men and women of other ethnic groups. If the enormous costs associated with osteoporotic fractures are to be reduced, the underlying problem must be designated as a disease so to allow maximal awareness and early detection, effective treatment, and long-term control.

HORMONAL REPLACEMENT THERAPY

On July 9, 2002, the National Institutes of Health dropped a bombshell. It terminated the Woman's Health Initiative Study[15] prematurely because the adverse effects of estrogen/progesterone replacement therapy (breast cancer, heart attack, blood clots, stroke) outweighed the benefits. At the time six million women, more or less, were taking hormonal therapy for a variety of reasons, the most common of which was osteoporosis.[16] Originally, in the 1960s, estrogen replacement therapy had been introduced for the relief of postmenopausal symptoms. The inference was that the medication should be used for a few months or, at most, for a year or two.

Gradually, hormonal replacement therapy gained in popularity.[17] In the 1970s, though, concern arose regarding the increased incidence of uterine cancer with estrogen use.[18] And soon thereafter, hormonal replacement therapy was noted to cause blood clots in the legs, lungs, and elsewhere.[19]

In the mid-1990s concern was raised regarding the effect of

estrogen therapy on breast tissue and the development of breast cancer.[20] So the results of the Woman's Health Initiative should not have been a surprise to those knowledgeable of the particulars relating to hormonal therapy. Most of the studies during the past thirty years that had shown beneficial effects from estrogenic hormones of one type or another were either retrospective, observational, or case-controlled. Such studies are open to biases, including some that were not recognized at the time of the study design. The only way to determine with any degree of certainty if estrogenic hormonal therapy is responsible for an effect of one type or another was to conduct a prospective, randomized, placebo-controlled trial. That was the rationale for the Woman's Health Initiative at commencement in 1993. It was meant to provide ultimate proof.

The study unearthed, as each year passed, a distressing array of side effects: (1) a 26 percent increase in breast cancer (when compared to the placebo group), (2) a 29 percent increase in heart attack, (3) a 100 percent increase in blood clots, and (4) a 41 percent increase in stroke. The conclusion was that whatever might be the benefit provided to those with osteoporosis, the side effects were an unacceptable risk.

A few months later, in May 2003, the Women's Health Initiative researchers had a second devastating announcement: The participants who had received hormonal replacement therapy were found to have a greater incidence of dementia (Alzheimer's disease)[21] than those who had received a placebo. The increased risk amounted to an additional twenty-three cases of dementia per ten thousand women per year. Earlier studies[22] that were later realized to have been poorly designed had suggested an opposite effect for hormonal replacement therapy.

Estrogen had been introduced in the 1950s at a time when the safety of a particular medical regimen was not subjected to the rigorous testing of today. The practice of medicine was more an art than a science. Today, the indications for a medication must be established on facts that have been quantified, reproduced, and subjected to rigorous testing. Science is now the foundation of medicine, and much more so than fifty years ago.

The women in the Women's Health Initiative trial did experience 24 percent fewer fractures than the control group. Such an effect had been demonstrated in prior clinical studies,[23] but the methodology employed during those trials had been questioned by some. The Women's Health Initiative study confirmed unequivocally those earlier results as they pertain to bone fracture. Now, though, because of the documented side effects, the rationale for estrogenic replacement therapy for osteoporosis has undergone a dramatic shift. Pharmaceutical research must be directed to drugs that will provide an effective treatment of osteoporosis without an adverse effect on the breast and on cardiovascular function. Stay tuned.

MAINTAINING SKELETAL INTEGRITY

When one considers the evidence taken as a whole, osteoporosis should be considered to be much less a target for hormonal therapy and much more a problem that can be arrested by dietary regimen and exercise. Both dietary calcium deficiency and sodium excess have been shown in well-conducted studies to be significant contributors to bone deterioration in the elderly.[24] And, more recently, animal protein, when consumed in excess, has become an established suspect.

Calcium lack in animals such as cats, rodents, and dogs causes osteoporosis.[25] Calcium balance studies in patients with osteoporosis have consistently demonstrated a negative calcium balance, with dietary calcium intake insufficient to account for calcium loss in the feces, urine, and perspiration.[26] Despite the number of studies that have addressed the issue of dietary calcium deficiency, there has been uncertainty and disagreement regarding how much calcium should be considered the minimal daily requirement. Recently, though, with the 1994 Consensus Development Conference on Optimal Calcium Intake, much of the confusion has been resolved. Briefly stated, the Consensus panel of the National Institutes of Health recommends a calcium intake of 1200–1500 mg/day for adolescents, 1000 mg/day for men up to age sixty-five, 1500 mg/day for postmenopausal women, and 1500 mg/day for everyone above age sixty-five.[27]

CALCIUM INTAKE

Calcium was abundant in the environment in which primitive humans evolved. Edible foliage, tubers, nuts, and other plant food available to herbivorous and omnivorous mammals have a relatively high calcium content[28] as a result of absorption from the soil by the root system of the plant.

Analysis of foods consumed by chimpanzees, our closest primate relatives, indicates that their diet has a high calcium content.[29] Studies of primitive societies in South Africa have shown that their diet is also very high in calcium. By way of contrast, today's diet in urbanized or industrialized nations commonly contains 600–650 mg/day of calcium or lower.[30]

Cereals are a big contributor to the calcium deficiency in the contemporary diet.[31] During the modern-day processing of grains, calcium is eliminated with the result that the refined breakfast product of today is low in calcium.

CALCIUM AND OSTEOPOROSIS

Recent studies have shown a positive effect of dietary calcium supplementation in preventing bone loss.[32] In one of the studies, the bone density at twelve sites was monitored in forty-four postmenopausal women and thirty controls. A significant salutary effect was shown for a 700 mg calcium supplement during the two-year observation period.

Hip fracture studies have been particularly enlightening. In Yugoslavia the incidence of hip fracture was 50 percent less in women from a community whose dietary calcium was about 1000 mg/day in comparison to the incidence for women in a community with half that amount.[33] And in a prospective study, a group of North Carolina researchers found a 60 percent lower hip fracture rate in both men and women in the upper third of calcium intake (over 765 mg/day) than in those in the lower third (below 470 mg/day).[34]

SODIUM, CALCIUM, AND OSTEOPOROSIS

Generally speaking, the diet of urbanized and industrialized societies contains an excessive amount of sodium. The excess is of such a degree that calcium is not processed properly as it passes through the kidney and, as a result, is lost into the urine along with the sodium. The calcium balance for the body becomes negative and calcium is resorbed from the skeleton on a continuing basis to maintain the proper calcium level within blood.[35]

In particular regard to postmenopausal women, the effect of sodium excess on urine calcium has been determined. Urinary calcium excretion increases, at the very least, by 10.5 mg per 1000 mg of incremental dietary sodium[36] (fig. 6), an amount that is less by 60

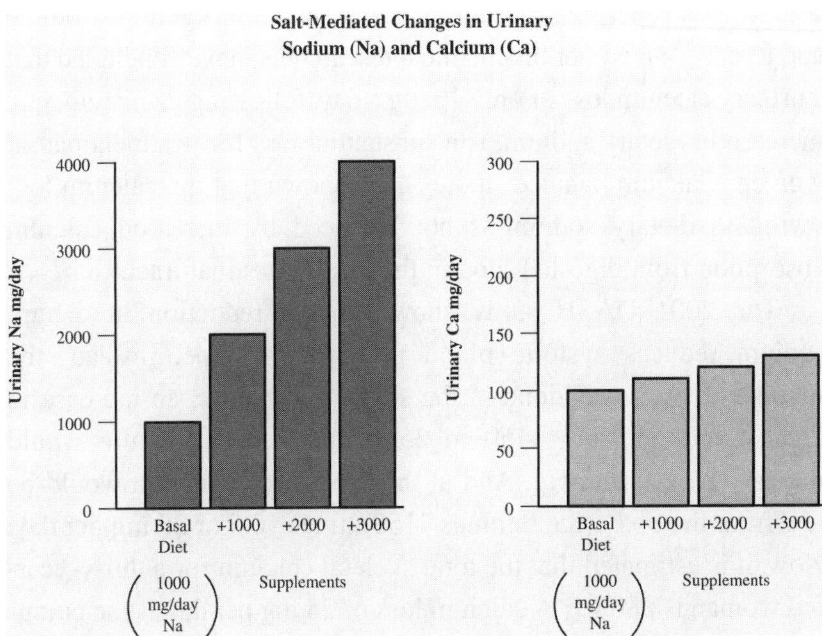

Fig. 6. Bar graph depicting salt-mediated changes in urinary sodium (Na) and calcium (Ca). **Left:** At a basal diet level of 1000 mg Na (the horizontal axis), the kidneys excrete 1000 mg of Na per day (the vertical axis). The body does not store sodium. As sodium is increased in the diet (salt supplements, on the horizontal axis), the kidneys promptly excrete that same amount, as reflected by the incremental size of the bars (on the vertical axis).

Right: A constant dietary intake is maintained. At the basal dietary level of 1000 mg of sodium per day, the kidney excretion of calcium for purposes of this depiction is 100 mg per day (the vertical axis). As sodium is supplemented to the diet, urinary calcium excretion increases. The calcium loss is 10.5 mg per 1000 mg of Na supplementation despite maintenance of a constant dietary intake of calcium. (Amended and reproduced with permission from the *British Medical Journal* 1989;**299**:834–835)

percent than the 25 mg value obtained by Sabto in an earlier study involving normal male subjects.[37] Nordin's conclusion that "100 mmol of sodium takes out 1 mmol of calcium" (in biochemical terminology)[38] is an easy relationship to remember and indicates a somewhat steeper relationship than that shown in figure 6. Both he and Evans,[39] and other biochemical researchers, have concluded that a urinary calcium loss of only 10 mg a day, following an incremental increase in dietary sodium, is a substantial loss for postmenopausal women. Calcium balance studies have shown that the calcium loss owing to dietary sodium is not balanced by increased calcium absorption from digested food in the gastrointestinal tract.

The 2001 DASH study shows how a reduction in dietary sodium reduces systolic blood pressure. Assume, instead, the reverse of what was done in the study, and that is, an increase in dietary sodium from 1150 to 3500 mg. Blood pressure would increase by 8.9 mm Hg. And at the same time, calcium would be lost from the body (3500 minus 1150) times 10.5 or 25 mg per day. Now, it is estimated that the total skeletal calcium for a thirty-year-old woman is 880 g.[40] A calcium loss of 25 mg per day is the cumulative equivalent of 8.8 g, or 1 percent total bone loss per year, assuming that the adaption to the dietary sodium took place solely as a result of bone resorption. A 1 percent loss of bone mass per year corresponds to the average skeletal deterioration sustained by many postmenopausal white women. Researchers have concluded that dietary sodium has an extraordinary effect on the development of postmenopausal osteoporosis[41] and that the effect can be totally offset by decreasing dietary sodium from the present 3500 mg (national average) to 1150.

The amount of calcium necessary to protect the skeleton and supply other needs of the body depends on the amount of sodium that individual is consuming. With greater sodium intake, more calcium is required. In one extraordinary study, during which bone density was determined at intervals during a two-year period of study (of 124 postmenopausal women) at the University of Western Australia,[42] bone loss was prevented, as determined by dual energy densitometry of a hip site, when sodium excretion was reduced to an average value of 2110 mg/day or lower (from a baseline value of 2783 mg/day) and at the same time, calcium intake was increased to 1768 mg or greater.

In other words, whenever sodium intake is greater than 2110 mg/day, calcium intake must be greater than 1768 mg/day in order to protect against bone loss. That amount of calcium dietary intake (something in excess of 1768 mg) is a theoretical value that would be very difficult, if not impossible, to achieve by diet. The authors also found that whenever calcium intake is reduced below 1768 mg/day, sodium intake must be less than 2100 mg. Thus, sodium has a profound effect on urinary calcium excretion and, for all practical purposes, must be kept below 2110 mg/day in order to prevent bone loss.

The relation between dietary calcium intake and urinary sodium excretion, determined by regression equation and maintenance of that change at zero (i.e., no bone loss), is shown in figure 7.

Other Factors That Influence Osteoporosis

Older studies have shown that tobacco usage,[43] alcoholism,[44] and coffee intake greater than four cups per day[45] are associated with increased propensity for osteoporosis.

Inadequate sunlight is another risk factor for osteoporosis. Inadequate sunlight exposure causes decreased formation of vitamin D, which in turn causes decreased calcium absorption from the intestine. The importance of marginal vitamin D deficiency in the pathogenesis of osteopenia with aging is of particular concern in Scandinavian countries where sunlight exposure is less during the calendar year.[46]

Obesity is protective. Immobilization, and even lack of physical exercise, predisposes people to bone loss.[47] In young healthy people bone mass is directly related to lean muscle mass and body

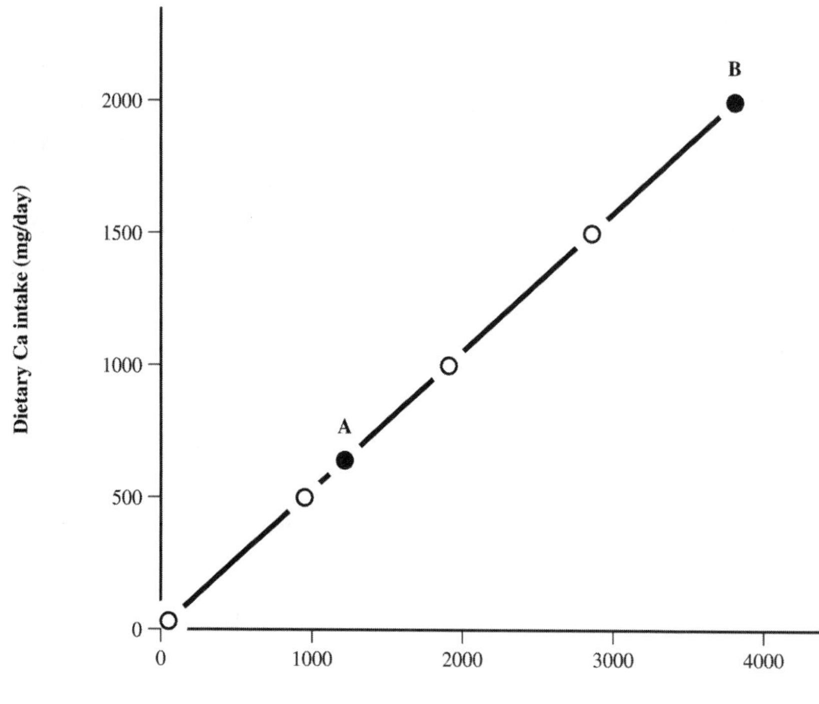

Fig. 7. The plot shows the relative amounts of dietary sodium and calcium required to maintain total hip bone density gained by multiple regression analysis. The influence of urinary sodium excretion and dietary calcium intake was examined in a two-year longitudinal study of 124 postmenopausal women. Neither habitual sodium intake or protein consumption (which averaged 72 grams/day) were manipulated during the study.

The study showed that both dietary calcium and dietary sodium are strong and significant determinants of bone mass. The amount of dietary calcium required to neutralize the effects of dietary sodium intake can be determined from the plot. For example, a calcium intake of 640 mg with a sodium excretion of 1200 mg (point A) would prevent bone loss. As daily sodium excretion (dietary sodium intake) increases to 4000 mg, calcium consumption must approach 2000 mg (point B). (Reproduced with permission by the *American Journal of Clinical Nutrition* 1995;**62**:740–745, American Society for Clinical Nutrition) size. The importance of physical exercise and maintenance of muscle mass is supported by many studies showing that regular physical exercise has a beneficial effect on bone mass.[48]

PROTEIN AND OSTEOPOROSIS

Evidence is accumulating that dietary protein is capable of causing bone loss and osteoporosis. In a well-controlled clinical trial, Sebastian[49] et al. showed, in a short-term analysis, that bone turnover in postmenopausal women resulted from mobilization of skeletal calcium salts used to balance acid from dietary protein intake. And in another equally impressive trial involving postmenopausal women,[50] an increased risk of osteoporotic forearm fractures was found with higher protein consumption. Of course, inadequate protein can have adverse effects, too.[51] But the evidence does indicate that abundant dietary protein can be harmful in older persons.[52]

The bottom line: A daily incremental increase in animal protein (meat, cheese, and the like) of 40 g increases urine calcium by 40 mg, which is a very significant amount. (See fig. 6 in chapter 7.)

ALTERNATIVE MEDICATION

The days of a paternalistic approach to osteoporosis care are over. The hormonal replacement therapy (HRT) episode will surely mean that women with osteoporosis will demand wider information regarding treatment options and associated risk factors. Women placed their trust in the medical and pharmaceutical professions when they accepted HRT; it is now the responsibility of those two professions to help them make informed decisions.

As it appears now, women concerned with osteoporosis might

be better served by tissue-specific estrogen compounds such as raloxifene,[53] a compound that possesses estrogen-like effects on bone but does not stimulate the breast. Raloxifene has already been shown to reduce fracture risk in a study where both the interventional group and the control group received calcium.[54] The effect for the raloxifene group developed in addition to the beneficial contribution of calcium.

Another alternative medication is a group called *biophosphonates*, which are potent inhibitors of bone resorption.[55]

ATTITUDE OF THE SALT INSTITUTE

The Salt Institute statement regarding osteoporosis begins as follows: "While few would dispute the positive relationship between dietary sodium intake and calcium excretion, the relative amounts of dietary sodium that would need to be eliminated for a paltry reduction in urinary calcium excretion has convinced most experts that the better dietary strategy is to promote increased intake of dairy products, not reduce dietary sodium."[56]

One might ask of the Salt Institute, who are the "most experts" to whom you refer? A review of medical literature for the past two decades shows that researchers have become increasingly concerned not only about the inadequacy of calcium intake for the maintenance of bone health but also about the effects of excessive dietary sodium on bone mineralization. The Salt Institute needs only to consider the facts. In Devine's University of Western Australia study (fig. 7), both dietary calcium and urinary sodium excretion were found to be powerful determinants of bone loss. When dietary sodium intake, as monitored by urinary excretion, approaches 4000 mg/day—an amount that is easily exceeded by patronage at fast-food outlets—calcium intake necessary to maintain an unchanged bone mass was found to be 2000 mg/day. The latter is a formidable amount when compared to the 642 mg/day average intake for present-day US adults. At the 642 mg calcium level, dietary sodium must be reduced to 1200 mgm to prevent loss (fig. 7). That amount, the Salt Institute should note, is considerably less than the US daily sodium consumption estimate of 3500 mg. So much more than the promotion of dairy products, as the Salt Institute recommends, is needed to maintain bone mass.

DAIRY PRODUCTS

Cheese is touted by the dairy industry (Dairy Management Incorporated) and its public relations arm, the National Dairy Council, for the prevention/treatment of osteoporosis, but clinical studies suggest a degree of caution. The problem is: Cheese is high in sodium (200 to 400 mg per ounce often), in protein (often 40 percent of total calories), and in fat (usually 55 percent of calories). The calcium in cheese is nice, but the sodium, the protein, and the fat are not. What's more, cheese contains densely packed calories and no vitamins and fiber. And who is not worried about the nutrient value of cheese? Well, Kraft Foods, the largest US producer of cheese products, is not. For good bone health they promote macaroni and cheese, frozen pizza, and the like. Is that not amazing? Do they really think that the public is so gullible as to believe cheese could be effective in the prevention of osteoporosis?

All of which brings up the subject of nutritional guidance. The Physicians Committee for Responsible Medicine (PCRM) has pointed out that the profit motive of the dairy industry interferes with its perception of nutritional problems. The self-stated interest of Dairy Management Incorporated is, as the PCRM emphasizes,[57] to "increase the output of dairy products on behalf of American dairy farmers."

Such statements by the PCRM rankle the dairy industry. In a press release response the National Dairy Council countered the PCRM criticism with some of its own: "Consumers are warned against taking nutritional guidance from activist groups [such as the PCRM]."

With a knee-jerk-like response to the Dairy Council remarks, the PCRM scored a point with the following return volley: "But isn't it much more hazardous for consumers to take nutritional guidance from business groups that are trying to promote their own agenda?"

While cheese is of questionable value in the prevention of osteoporosis, milk and other low-fat dairy products contain much calcium and can be expected to provide a protective effect. But the value of milk is not conceded by all researchers. For instance, in one prospective analysis, the Harvard Nurses' Health Study, during which 77,761 nurses were followed for twelve years, no protective effect was noted from increased milk consumption on fracture risk.[58] Those who drank three or more glasses of milk per day, a goal that is prescribed by the Dairy Council, had no reduction at all in the risk of hip or arm fracture compared with women who did not consume any dairy products. In fact, the fracture rate was higher for those who consumed three plus servings in comparison to those who did not drink milk. An Australian study showed similar results.[59] But one can substantially decrease the risk of osteoporosis by reducing sodium and animal protein and increasing calcium in the diet,[60] by increasing intake of fruits and vegetables,[61] and by maintaining an active lifestyle.[62]

It is to be realized that dairy products are not the only source of calcium. Consider that the original source of calcium is in the ground. Calcium, and other minerals, are dissolved in watery solutes and are absorbed into plants by way of the roots. The minerals become incorporated into the stems, leaves, flowers, and fruits of plants. Humans can get plenty of calcium the same way that cows do—from edible plant foods. So a cup of spinach leaves contains 244 mg Ca, an orange

56 mg, and a cup of navy beans 128 mg. Fruit, vegetables, and low-fat diary products supply one with ample amounts of dietary calcium that, when combined with the avoidance of dietary sodium and excessive dietary protein, will truly prevent bone loss as we age.

INTERNET

Google lists sixteen million entries for osteoporosis, but readers who search those sites will find only limited help. For instance, Google's number one osteoporosis listing, the United States' National Osteoporosis Foundation (NOF), which describes itself as the nation's leading voluntary health organization solely directed to osteoporosis and bone health (see www.nof.org), fails to include dietary restriction of sodium and animal protein among preventative measures. Instead, the NOF lists only the following among the five steps needed for good bone health:

1. Calcium and vitamin D
2. Weight-bearing exercise
3. Abstinence from smoking and excessive alcohol
4. Conversation with one's doctor regarding bone health
5. Bone density testing and medication when appropriate

And what about sodium and protein excess? Inscrutably, there is no mention of those two important determinants of bone health.

Along the way, in the scroll through Google's entries, avoid the NIH ORBD-NRC—Osteoporosis Overview listing. As recently as June 2005, the material for that site had not been revised since October 2000. So estrogen replacement therapy was still being recommended for maintenance of bone density in postmenopausal women and erroneous statements were still being put forward regarding a supposed salutary effect of supplemental estrogen on the heart. The Web site needs to include information from the July 2002 Women's Health Initiative hormone replacement study in its updated material.

Finally, some worthwhile information emerges at the Welcome to Osteoporosis Australia site (www.osteoporosis.org.au). Osteoporosis Australia, an independent consumer and health professional organization, emphasizes that good bone health requires salt and animal protein restriction in the diet. And that's what much be said.

NOTES

The author's grateful acknowledgment: Professor B. E. C. Nordin of the Institute of Medicine and Veterinary Science in Adelaide, Australia, reviewed this chapter and provided numerous helpful suggestions.

1. Gutin, BKM. Can vigorous exercise play a role in osteoporosis prevention? a review. *Osteoporosis International* 1992;**2**:55–69.

2. Mundy, GR. Bone remolding of bone loss in osteoporosis. In: *Osteoporosis: Diagnosis and Management.* Meunier, PJ (ed.). Martin Dunitz Ltd. 1998, pp. 17–35.

3. Mazess, RB. On aging bone loss. *Clinical Orthopaedics & Related Research* 1982;**165**:239–252.

Riggs, BL et al. Differential changes in bone mineral density of the appendicular and axial skeleton with aging: relationship to spinal osteoporosis. *Journal of Clinical Investigations* 1981;**67**:328–335.

Smith, DM and Khairi, MRA and Johnston, CC Jr. The loss of bone mineral with aging and its relationship to risk of fracture. *Journal of Clinical Investigation* 1975;**56**:311–318.

4. Trotter, ML et al. Densities of bones of white and negro skeletons. *Journal of Bone and Joint Surgery* (Am) 1960;**42**:50–58.

5. Bauer, RL. Ethnic differences in hip fracture in Bexar County. *Journal of Clinical Research* 1986;**34**:358.

6. Ross, PD et al. A comparison of hip fracture incidence among native Japanese, Japanese Americans, and American Caucasians. *American Journal of Epidemiology* 1991;**133**:801–809.

7. Kanis, JA and WHO Study Group. Assessment of fracture risk and its application for screening for postmenopausal osteoporosis: synopsis of a WHO report. *Osteoporosis International* 1994;**4**:368–381.

Kanis, JA et al. The diagnosis of osteoporosis. *Journal of Bone and Mineral Research* 1994;**9**:1137–1141.

One standard deviation away from the mean in either direction on the horizontal axis for a bell-shaped curve accounts for around 68 percent of the grouping; 2.5 standard deviations away from the mean accounts for roughly 98 percent of the grouping. See http://www.geographyfieldwork.com/StandardDeviation for complete explanation.

8. Ibid.

9. Ibid.

10. Melton, LJ III et al. How many women have osteoporosis now? *Journal of Bone and Mineral Research* 1992;**7**:1005–1010.

11. Melton, LJ III. How many women have osteoporosis now? *Journal of Bone and Mineral Research* 1995;**10**:175–177.

12. Melton, LJ III et al. How many women have osteoporosis now? *Journal of Bone and Mineral Research* 1992;**7**:1005–1010.

13. Melton, LJ III. How many women have osteoporosis now? *Journal of Bone and Mineral Research* 1995;**10**:175–177.

14. Phillips, SJ et al. A community blood pressure survey: Rochester, Minnesota, 1986. *Mayo Clinic Proceedings* 1988;**63**:691–699.

15. Writing Group for the Women's Health Initiative Investigators. Risks and benefits of estrogen plus progestin in healthy postmenopausal women, principal results from the Women's Health Initiative randomized controlled trial. *JAMA* 2002;**288**:321–333. The report came shortly after the publication of the results of the Heart Estrogen/Progestin Replacement Study (HERS) in an earlier 2002 issue of the *JAMA*, a study which documented substantial risk with hormonal replacement therapy, and at the same time of another study which documented, in the *JAMA*, an increased risk of ovarian cancer in patients taking estrogen alone.

16. Felson, DT et al. The effect of postmenopausal estrogen therapy on bone density in elderly women. *New England Journal of Medicine* 1993;**329**:1141–1146.

17. By the mid-1990s studies had appeared that advocated the consideration of hormonal replacement therapy for heart disease (Gradstein, F et al. Postmenopausal estrogen and progestin use and the risk of cardiovascular disease. *New England Journal of Medicine* 1996;**335**:453–461. Also Henderson, BE et al. Estrogen use and cardiovascular disease. *American Journal of Obstetrics and Gynecology* 1986;**154**:1181–1186) and, even, for Alzheimer's disease (Tang, MX et al. Effect of estrogen during menopause on risk and age of onset of Alzheimer's disease. *The Lancet* 1996;**348**:429–432).

18. Ziel, HK and Finkle, WD. Increased risk of endometrial carcinoma among users of conjugated estrogens. *New England Journal of Medicine* 1975;**293**:1167–1170.

19. Gradstein, E et al. Prospective study of exogenous hormones and risk of pulmonary embolism in women. *The Lancet* 1996;**348**:983–987.

20. Colditz, GA et al. The use of estrogens and progestins and the risk of breast cancer in postmenopausal women. *New England Journal of Medicine* 1995;**332**:1589–1593.

21. Shumaker, SA et al. Estrogen plus progestin and the incidence of dementia and mild cognitive impairment in postmenopausal women: the Women's Health Initiative Memory Study: a randomized controlled trial. *JAMA* 2003;**289**:2651–2662.

22. Kawas, C et al. A prospective study of estrogen replacement therapy and the risk of developing Alzheimer disease: the Baltimore Longitudinal Study on Aging. *Neurology* 1997;**48**:1517–1521.

Yaffe, K, et al. Estrogen therapy in postmenopausal women: effects on cognitive function and dementia. *JAMA* 1998;**279**:688–695.

23. Cauley, JA et al. Estrogen replacement therapy and fractures in older women. *Annals Internal Medicine* 1995;**122**:9–16.

24. Itoh, R et al. Dietary sodium, an independent determinant for urinary deoxypyridinoline in elderly women. A cross-sectional study on the effect of dietary factors on deoxypyridinole excretion in 12-h urine spec-

imens from 763 free-living Japanese. *European Journal of Clinical Nutrition* 1999;**53**:886–890.

Devine, A et al. A longitudinal study of the effect of sodium and calcium intakes on regional bone density in postmenopausal women. *American Journal of Clinical Nutrition* 1995;**62**:740–745.

Nordin, BE Christopher and Heaney, RP. Calcium supplementation of the diet: justified by present evidence. *British Medical Journal* 1990;**300**:1056–1060.

Heaney, RP et al. Calcium nutrition and bone health in the elderly. *American Journal of Clinical Nutrition* 1982;**36**:986–1013.

25. Ammann, P et al. Preclinical evaluation of new therapeutic agents for osteoporosis. In: *Osteoporosis: Diagnosis and Management.* Meunier, PJ (ed.). St. Louis: Mosby, 1998, pp. 257–273.

Gold, E and Goulding, A. High dietary salt intakes lower bone mineral density in ovariectomised rats: a dual x-ray absorptiometry study. *Bone* 1995;**16**:1S, 115S (abstr).

26. Matkovic, V et al. Bone status and fracture rates in two regions of Yugoslavia. *American Journal of Clinical Nutrition* 1979;**32**:540–549.

Nilas, L and Christiansen, C and Rodbro, P. Calcium supplementation and postmenopausal bone loss. *British Medical Journal* 1984;**289**:1103–1106.

Freudenheim, JL and Johnson, NE and Smith, EL. Relationships between usual nutrient intake and bone-mineral content of women 35–65 years of age: longitudinal and cross-sectional analysis. *American Journal of Clinical Nutrition* 1986;**44**:863–876.

Dawson-Hughes, B and Jacques, P and Shipp, C. Dietary calcium intake and bone loss from the spine in healthy postmenopausal women. *American Journal of Clinical Nutrition* 1987;**46**:685–687.

Riggs, BL et al. Dietary calcium intake and rates of bone loss in women. *Journal of Clinical Investigation* 1987;**80**:979–982.

27. NIH Consensus Conference. Optimal calcium intake. *JAMA* 1994;**272**:1942–1948.

28. Eaton, SB and Konner, M. Paleolithic Nutrition. A consideration of its nature and current implications. *New England Journal of Medicine* 1985;**315**:283–289.

Eaton and Bond and Nelson, DA. Calcium in evolutionary perspective. *American Journal of Clinical Nutrition* 1991;**54**:2815–2875.

Cordan, L et al. Plant-animal subsistence ratios and macronutrient energy estimates in worldwide hunter-gatherers diets. *American Journal of Clinical Nutrition* 2000;**71**:682–692.

29. Wehmeyer, AS et al. The nutrient composition and dietary importance of some vegetable foods eaten by Kung Bushman. *South African Medical Journal* 1969;**40**:1529–1530.

30. Euronut Seneea Investigators: Cruz, AA et al. Intake of vitamins and minerals. *European Journal of Clinical Nutrition* 1990;**45(Suppl 3)**:121–138.

Chapuy, MC et al. Vitamin D3 and calcium to prevent hip fractures in elderly women. *New England Journal of Medicine* 1993;**237**:1637–1642.

31. Eaton, SB and Konner, M. Paleolithic Nutrition. A consideration of its nature and current implications. *New England Journal of Medicine* 1985;**315**:283–289.

Eaton and Bond and Nelson, DA. Calcium in evolutionary perspective. *American Journal of Clinical Nutrition* 1991;**54**:2815–2875.

Cordan, L et al. Plant-animal subsistence ratios and macronutrient energy estimates in worldwide hunter-gatherers diets. *American Journal of Clinical Nutrition* 2000;**71**:682–692.

32. Uusi-Rasi, K et al. Changes in bone mineral density during a mean 4-year follow-up. In: *Nutritional Aspects of Osteoporosis*. Burckhardt, P and Dawson-Hughes, B and Heaney, R (eds.). San Diego: Academic Press, 2001, pp. 65–74.

Dawson-Hughes, B et al. Effect of calcium and vitamin D supplementation on bone density in men and women 65 years of age or older. *New England Journal of Medicine* 1997;**337**:670–676.

Cumming, RG and Nevitt, MC. Calcium for prevention of osteoporotic fractures in postmenopausal women. *Journal of Bone and Mineral Research* 1997;**12**:1321–1329.

Seeman, E et al. Risk Factors for Osteoporosis in Men. *American Journal of Medicine* 1983;**75**:977–982.

33. Matkowic, V et al. Bone status and fracture rates in two regions of Yugoslavia. *American Journal of Clinical Nutrition* 1979;**32**:540–549.

34. Holbrook, TL and Barrett-Connor, E and Wingard, D. Dietary calcium and risk of hip fracture. *The Lancet* 1988;**ii**:1046–1049.

35. Breslau, NA et al. The role of dietary sodium of renal excretion and intestinal adsorption of calcium and on vitamin D metabolism. *Journal of Clinical Endocrinology & Metabolism* 1982;**55**: 369–373.

Nordin, BE et al. The nature and significance of the relationship between urinary sodium and urinary calcium in women. *Journal of Nutrition* 1993;**123**:1615–1622.

Matkovic, V et al. Urinary calcium, sodium, and bone mass of young females. *American Journal of Clinical Nutrition* 1995;**62**:417–425.

Evans, CEL et al. The effect of dietary sodium on calcium metabolism in premenopausal and postmenopausal women. *European Journal of Clinical Nutrition* 1997;**51**:394–399.

36. McParland, BE and Goulding, A and Campbell, AJ. Dietary salt affects biochemical markers of resorption and formation of bone in elderly women. *British Medical Journal* 1989;**299**:834–835.

Zarkadas, M et al. Sodium chloride supplementation and urinary calcium excretion in postmenopausal women. *American Journal of Clinical Nutrition* 1989;**50**:1088–1094.

37. Sabto, et al. Influence of urinary sodium on calcium excretion in normal individuals. *Medical Journal of Australia* 1984;**140**:354–356.

38. Ibid.

39. Breslau, NA et al. The role of dietary sodium of renal excretion and intestinal adsorption of calcium and on vitamin D metabolism. *Journal of Clinical Endocrinology & Metabolism* 1982;**55**:369–373.

Nordin, BE et al. The nature and significance of the relationship between urinary sodium and urinary calcium in women. *Journal of Nutrition* 1993;**123**:1615–1622.

Matkovic, V et al. Urinary calcium, sodium, and bone mass of young females. *American Journal of Clinical Nutrition* 1995;**62**:417–425.

Evans, CEL et al. The effect of dietary sodium on calcium metabolism in premenopausal and postmenopausal women. *European Journal of Clinical Nutrition* 1997;**51**:394–399.

40. Riggs, BL et al. Differential changes in bone mineral density of the appendicular and axial skeleton with aging: relationship to spinal osteoporosis. *Journal of Clinical Investigation* 1981;**67**:328–335.

41. Breslau, NA et al. The role of dietary sodium of renal excretion and intestinal adsorption of calcium and on vitamin D metabolism. *Journal of Clinical Endocrinology & Metabolism* 1982;**55**: 369–373.

Nordin, BE et al. The nature and significance of the relationship between urinary sodium and urinary calcium in women. *Journal of Nutrition* 1993;**123**:1615–1622.

Matkovic, V et al. Urinary calcium, sodium, and bone mass of young females. *American Journal of Clinical Nutrition* 1995;**62**:417–425.

Evans, CEL et al. The effect of dietary sodium on calcium metabolism in premenopausal and postmenopausal women. *European Journal of Clinical Nutrition* 1997;**51**:394–399.

42. Itoh, R et al. Dietary sodium, an independent determinant for urinary deoxypyridinoline in elderly women. A cross-sectional study on the effect of dietary factors on deoxypyridinole excretion in 12-h urine specimens from 763 free-living Japanese. *European Journal of Clinical Nutrition* 1999;**53**:886–890.

Devine, A et al. A longitudinal study of the effect of sodium and calcium intakes on regional bone density in postmenopausal women. *American Journal of Clinical Nutrition* 1995;**62**:740–745.

Nordin, BE Christopher and Heaney, RP. Calcium supplementation of the diet: justified by present evidence. *British Medical Journal* 1990; **300**:1056–1060.

Heaney, RP et al. Calcium nutrition and bone health in the elderly. *American Journal of Clinical Nutrition* 1982;**36**:986–1013.

43. Daniell, HW. Osteoporosis of the slender smoker: vertebral compression fractures and loss of metacarpal cortex in relation to postmenopausal cigarette smoking and lack of obesity. *Archives of Internal Medicine* 1976;**136**:298–304.

44. Seeman, E et al. Risk factors for spinal osteoporosis in men. *American Journal of Medicine* 1983;**75**:977–983.

45. Cummings, SR et al. Risk factors for hip fracture in white women. *New England Journal of Medicine* 1995;**332**:776–773.

46. Heikinheimo, RJ et al. Annual injection of vitamin D and fractures of aged bones. *Calcified Tissue International* 1992;**51**:105–110.

47. Chalmers, J. Geographic variations in senile osteoporosis. The association with physical activity. *Journal of Bone and Joint Surgery* 1970;**52**:667–675.

48. Lüthje, P. Incidence of hip fracture in Finland: a forecast for 1990. *Acta Orthopaedic Scandinavica* 1985;**56**:223–225.

Mosekilde, L. Osteoporosis and exercise. *Bone* 1995;**17**:193–195.

White, MK et al. The effects of exercise on the bones of postmenopausal women. *International Orthopaedics* 1984;**7**:209–214.

Heinonen, A et al. Bone mineral density in female athletes representing sports with different loading characteristics of the skeleton. *Bone* 1995;**17**:197–203.

Leichter, I et al. Gain in mass density of bone following strenuous physical activity. *Journal of Orthopaedic Research* 1989;**7**:86–90.

49. Sebastian, A et al. Improved mineral balance and skeletal metabolism in postmenopausal women treated with potassium bicarbonate. *New England Journal of Medicine* 1994;**330**:1776–1781.

50. Feskanich, D et al. Protein consumption and bone fractures in women. *American Journal of Epidemiology* 1996;**143**:472–479.

51. Bonjour, JP and Sürch, MA and Rizzoli, R. Nutritional aspect of hip fractures. *Bone* 1996;**18**:139S–144S.

Bonjour, JP and Sürch, MA and Rizzoli, R. Proteins and bone health. *Pathological Biology (Paris)* 1997;**45**:57–59.

52. Barzel, US. The skeleton as an ion exchange system: implications for the role of acid-base imbalance in the genesis of osteoporosis. *Journal of Bone and Mineral Research* 1995;**10**:1431–1436.

Barzel, US, Massey, LK. Excess dietary protein can adversely affect bone. *Journal of Nutrition* 1998;**128**:1051–1053.

Williams, B et al. Metabolic acidosis and skeletal muscle adaptation to low protein diets in chronic uremia. *Kidney International* 1991;**40**:779–786.

53. Draper, MW et al. A controlled trial with raloxifene (LY139481)

HCl: impact on human bone turnover and serum lipid profile in healthy postmenopausal women. *Journal of Bone and Mineral Research* 1996;**11**:835–842.

54. Ettinger, B et al. Reduction of vertebral fracture risk in postmenopausal women with osteoporosis treated with raloxifene: results from a 3-year randomized clinical trial. *JAMA* 1999;**282**:637–645.

55. Reginster, JYL. Biophosphorates for the treatment of osteoporosis. In: *Osteoporosis: Diagnosis and Management.* Meunier, PJ (ed.). Martin Dunitz Ltd., 1998, pp. 123–130.

Reid, IR. Intravenous zoledronic acid in postmenopausal women with low bone mineral density. *New England Journal of Medicine* 2002;**346**:653–661.

56. http://www.saltinstitute.org/pubstat/who-4-02.html.

57. Physicians Committee for Responsible Medicine. Calcium, osteoporosis, and the selling of dairy products. http://www.makingpages.org/health/calcium.osteoporosis.html.

58. Feskanich, D et al. Milk, dietary calcium, and bone fractures in women: a 12 year prospective study. *American Journal of Public Health* 1997;**87**:992–997.

59. Cumming, RG and Klineberg, RJ. Case-controlled study of risk factors for hip fractures in the elderly. *American Journal of Epidemiology* 1994;**139**:493–505.

60. Finn, SC. The skeleton crew: is calcium enough? *Journal of Women's Health* 1998;**7(1)**:31–36.

Nordin, C. Calcium and osteoporosis. *Nutrition* 1997;**3(7/8)**:664–686.

Reid, DM and New, SA. Nutritional influences on bone mass. *Proceedings of the Nutrition Society* 1997;**56**:977–987.

61. Tucker, KL et al. Potassium, magnesium, and fruit and vegetable intakes are associated with greater bone mineral density in elderly men and women. *American Journal of Clinical Nutrition* 1999;**69**:727–736.

62. Prince, R et al. The effects of calcium supplementation (milk powder or tablets) and exercise on bone mineral density in postmenopausal women. *Journal of Bone and Mineral Research* 1995;**10**:1068–1075.

CHAPTER 9

DIETARY SODIUM—ADDITIONAL CONCERNS

CANCER OF THE STOMACH

Based upon an observation in 1965 that the death rate from stomach cancer, illustrated in figure 1, and stroke were strongly correlated and that the regression lines for each, over a two-decade period, were similar, the hypothesis has been presented[1] that salt could be involved in the etiology of each, though by different mechanisms. For stomach cancer it was postulated that high doses of salt causes injury to the inner wall of the stomach, thereby increasing the risk of cancer later on.

In the early 1990s, the hypothesis was expanded to include a bacterium, *Helicobacter pylori*.[2] It has been postulated that excessive use of dietary salt causes, over an extended period of time, injury to the acid-producing cells within the stomach. As the cellular population within the inner wall of the stomach decreases, the digestive juices of the stomach become less acidic. As a result, the

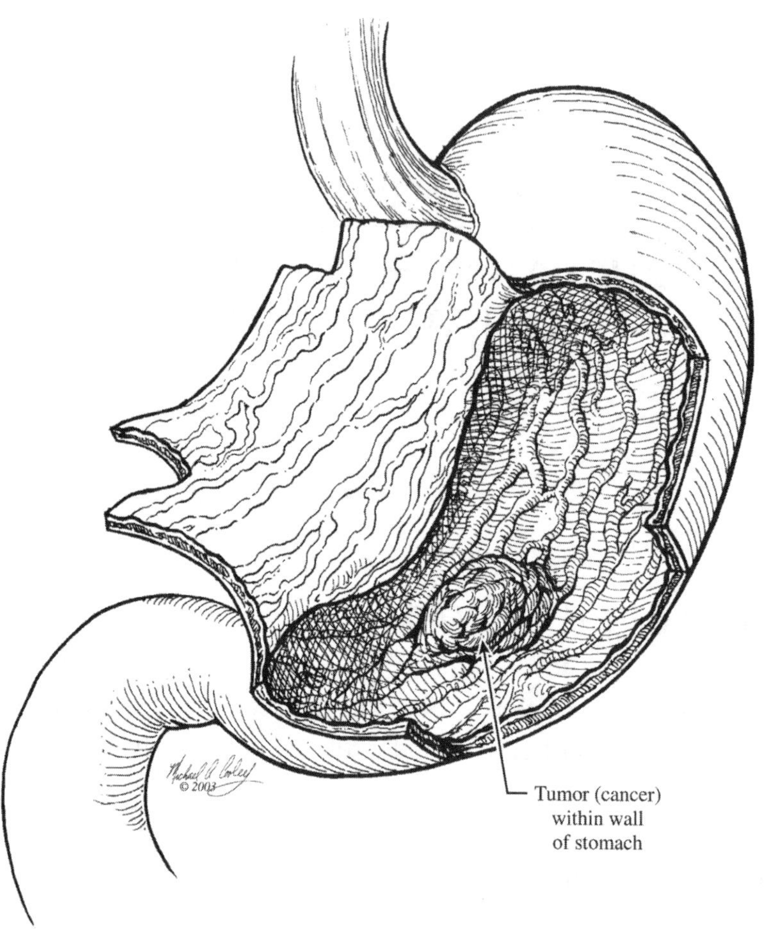

Fig. 1. Carcinoma (arrow) within lower portion of stomach. The polypoid lesion protrudes into the lumen of the stomach. Stomach carcinoma can also develop within an ulcer. A particularly devastating type of stomach cancer, scirrhous, infiltrates widely throughout the wall of the stomach.

bacterium *Helicobacter pylori* begins to thrive within the stomach juices. A bacterial invasion of such type favors the conversion of dietary nitrates, in cured and pickled products for instance, to cancer-causing nitrosamides and nitroamines.

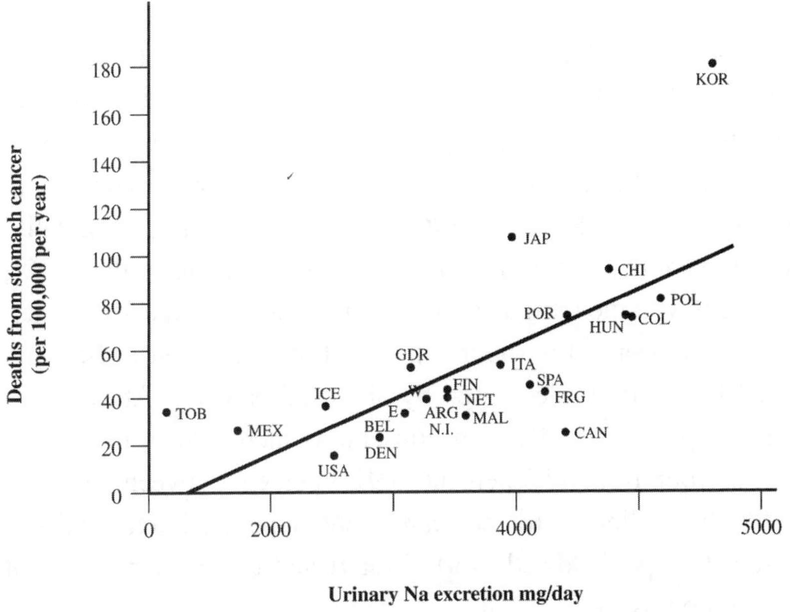

Fig. 2. The relation of urinary salt excretion and stomach cancer for men in twenty-four countries. $r = 0.70$, $p < 0.001$. (Reproduced with permission from Jooseens, JV et al. *International Journal of Epidemiology* 1996; **25**: 494–501. Oxford University Press)

In the mid-1990s the salt hypothesis gained further ground with the application of INTERSALT data to stomach cancer mortality rates.[3] The sodium excretion data that had been obtained from thirty-two countries worldwide during the INTERSALT trials were used for comparative regression analysis in respect to stomach cancer mortality rates. The relationship had a statistical significance of high degree (fig. 2).[4]

Refrigeration

During the latter half of the twentieth century, refrigeration became commonplace in the industrialized world, negating the necessity for using salt to prevent spoilage. During that same period of time, mortality from stomach cancer and stroke trended downward. In Japan only 9 percent of households had a refrigerator in 1960 versus 91 percent in 1970.[5] Urinary sodium was, on average, 6000 mg/day in 1955 for the people of Japan, and 4500 mg/day in 1987.[6] Researchers noted that both stomach cancer and stroke mortality in Japan started to decline in the 1960s, whereas both types of mortality declined significantly in the United States beginning in the 1930s, coincident with the introduction of refrigeration at that earlier time.[7]

Urinary twenty-four-hour salt excretion, measured in Belgium from 1966 to 1986, decreased by about 25 percent.[8] At the same time, refrigerators in Belgian households increased in the lowest income group from 37.5 percent to 91.3 percent between 1975 and 1985.[9] The decline in stomach cancer and hypertension mortality in western Europe followed World War II and the greater degree of refrigeration usage.

Mechanism for Stomach Cancer Development

It was 1993 when stomach cancer was found to be significantly related to the presence of a bacterium, *Helicobacter pylori*, that can be cultured from aspirated stomach juices. Analysis has shown that the prevalence of *H. pylori* in population samples is significantly correlated with salt intake levels for ten European countries.[10] On the basis of data gathered so far, *H. pylori* appears to be an operative risk factor only at higher salt intake values. The chain of events is thought to be as follows: Excessive dietary salt injuries the inner lining of the stomach following which *H. pylori* becomes established within the digestive juices. Then, potent nitromutagens and other cancer-forming chemicals tend to form within the stomach.[11]

American Cancer Society

The American Cancer Society has taken this position: "An increased risk of stomach cancer is associated with diets containing large amounts of smoked food, salted fish and meat, certain foods high in starch that are also low in fiber, and pickled vegetables." They have not taken a position condemning salt usage, however.[12]

Salt Institute

The Salt Institute has taken a position regarding salt usage and stomach cancer. They note that there are some "people who consume enormous amounts of salt-cured and pickled foods" and that "it is appropriate to direct a message to that subgroup." In other words: It is appropriate for health agencies, such as the American Cancer Society, to direct a message of caution to that subgroup. They go on to say that "it is totally inappropriate [on the other hand] to highlight that message and suggest that intakes in the 'safety hygienic range' of 1,200–4,600 or 5,750 mg/day sodium represents a concern for the general public or that cancer prevention demands reducing dietary sodium to 2,000 mg/day or less."[13] What they do not acknowledge, for the edification of the public, is that an association of dietary salt intake and stomach cancer has been uncovered, and what they do not explain is that while the frequency of stomach cancer has decreased greatly in recent decades, the parameters of the dietary salt/stomach cancer relationship have yet to be resolved. The concern, at this time, cannot be restricted to those who use enormous amounts of salt. It could be that a moderate amount of salt, consumed over an extended period of time, might have a carcinogenic effect on the stomach of a sensitive individual.

ASTHMA

Recent studies in humans have demonstrated a positive association between increased dietary salt consumption on bronchial reactivity and mortality from asthma.[14] The bronchioles are the tubular segments that carry inhaled air to the lung and excreted carbon dioxide in the reverse direction. Several experiments have shown that bronchial reactivity/irritability is increased as a result of a high-sodium diet.[15] Epidemiological studies in Wales and England have demonstrated an association between mortality from asthma and high sodium intake. The evidence is clearer for men than for women.

The most recent trial assessed the effects of dietary salt alteration in symptomatic asthma. The randomized study design was blinded to both the patient and the researcher and included a crossover period to an alternate regimen. The subjects were established on a low-sodium diet (1800 mg/day) and then randomized to receive 4500 mg/day or a matching placebo for five weeks.

Expiratory flow rates and bronchial responsiveness to methacholine challenge were recorded twice daily for each subject. The results of the study, conducted at Glenfield General Hospital in Leicester, England,[16] indicated that dietary sodium does exacerbate the severity of asthma in asthmatic patients. The authors concluded that the results were modest, nevertheless, and that sodium restriction as a therapeutic intervention is likely to be of use only in asthmatic patients with high daily sodium intake.

The mechanism by which sodium increases bronchial reactivity has not yet been elucidated. But animal experiments have shown that the hyperreactivity of sensitized bronchial smooth muscle is associated with an exaggerated influx of sodium across the cell membranes.[17]

The association between dietary salt and asthma may help to explain geographical variations in the prevalence of asthma and the rise in prevalence in underdeveloped countries as they adopt a Western lifestyle. Much more research needs to be done to unravel the mechanism of change resulting from dietary salt excess.

Salt Institute (continued)

The asthma-sodium relationship has not escaped the attention of the salt manufacturers. And, true to form, the medical reports that have been published to date were dismissed, summarily, by the Salt Institute in a report to the US Food and Nutrition Board:

> The quality of data that might be advanced to sustain a causal relationship of dietary salt and asthma does not merit . . . [your] attention. Asthma is a rampant health problem the understanding of which has been compromised by "experts" raising spurious issues. There has been no precipitous increase in children's salt intake.[18]

So, instead of carefully considering the merits of the science, the salt manufacturers protect their "turf" with an ostrichlike denial.

NOTES

1. Joossens, JV. La relation l'èpidèmiologie des accidentes cèrèbro-vasculaires et du cancer de l'estomac. *L'èvolution Mèdicale* 1968; **123**:381–385.

2. Tsuegane, S et al. *Helicobacter pylori*, dietary factors, and atrophic gastritis in five Japanese populations with different gastric cancer mortality. *Cancer Causes and Control* 1993;**4**:297–305.

The Eurogast Study Group. An international association between *Helicobacter pylori* infection and gastric cancer. *The Lancet* 1993; **341**:1359–1362.

3. Jooseens, JV et al. Dietary salt, nitrate and stomach cancer mortality in 24 countries. *International Journal of Epidemiology* 1996; **25**:494–501.

4. Shown for men only. The plot for women was slightly steeper (r = 0.74).

5. Hirayama, T. Epidemiology of stomach cancer in Japan. With special reference to the strategy for the primary prevention. *Japanese Journal of Clinical Oncology* 1984;**14**:159–168.

6. Sasaki, N. The relationship of salt intake to hypertension in the Japanese. *Geriatrics* 1964;**19**:735–744.

Cooperative Research Group. INTERSALT: an international study of electrolyte excretion and blood pressure. Results for 24 h urinary sodium and potassium excretion. *British Medical Journal* 1988;**297**:319–328.

7. Joossens, JV and Geboers, J. Epidemiology of gastric cancer: a clue to etiology. In: *Precancerous Lesions of the Gastrointestinal Tract.* Sherlock, P et al. (eds.). New York: Raven Press, 1993, pp. 97–113.

8. Joossens, JV and Kesteloot, H. Trends in systolic blood pressure, 24-hour sodium excretion, and stroke mortality in the elderly in Belgium. *American Journal of Medicine* 1991;(**Suppl. 3A**):5S–11S.

9. Joossens, JV and Kestloot, H. Community control of hypertension in Belgium: the role of nutrition. In: *Geriatric Hypertension.* Cuervo, CA and Robinson, BE and Sheppard, HL (eds.). Tampa: University of South Florida Press, 1989, pp. 157–189.

10. The Eurogast Study Group. An international association between *Helicobacter pylori* infection and gastric cancer. *The Lancet* 1993;**341**:1359–1362.

11. Jooseens, JV et al. Dietary salt, nitrate and stomach cancer mortality in 24 countries. *International Journal of Epidemiology* 1996;**25**:494–501.

12. http://www.cancer.org.

13. http://www.saltinstitute.org.

14. Carey, OJ et al. Effect of alterations of dietary sodium on the severity of asthma in men. *Thorax* 1993;**48**:714–718.

15. Burney, PGJ et al. Response to inhaled histamine and 24 hour sodium excretion. *British Medical Journal* 1986;**292**:1483–1486.

Burney, PGJ et al. Effect of changing dietary sodium on the airway response to histamine. *Thorax* 1989;**44**:36–41.

Javaid, A and Cushley, MJ and Bone, MF. Effect of dietary salt on bronchial reactivity to histamine in asthma. *British Medical Journal* 1988;**297**:454.

16. Carey, OJ et al. Effect of alterations of dietary sodium on the severity of asthma in men. *Thorax* 1993;**48**:714–718.

17. Souhrada, M and Souhrada, JF. Sensitisation induced sodium influxes in airway smooth muscle cells. *American Review of Respiratory Disease* 1985;**131**:A356.

18. http://www.saltinstitute.org/pubstat/fnb.html.

CHAPTER 10

WHAT IF IT'S ALL BEEN A BIG FAT LIE?

Will the information provided by the 1997 and 2001 DASH studies propel food-conscious consumers along the wrong pathway? Hardly. But that was the gist of a July 7, 2002, *New York Times Magazine* centerpiece story authored by Gary Taubes and entitled "What If It's All Been a Big Fat Lie?"[1]

In 1998 Taubes authored a report for the journal *Science*,[2] which faulted the 1997 DASH study. Four months later the article appeared on the Salt Institute Web site, where it remained for the next three years. The 1998 piece was far off the mark. Instead of critically reviewing the key aspect of the 1997 DASH study—the finding that adherence to a food pyramid anchored by fruits, vegetables, grain, and low-fat dairy products lowers blood pressure—Taubes directed his *Science* report to a tangential issue that appealed to his journalistic instincts more: dietary salt restriction. He assumed, incorrectly to be sure, that the 1997 report had restored the salt shaker to an honored position on the dining table.

Switch forward to July 2002 and the *New York Times* piece. Taubes directed his attention to the obesity and diabetes epidemic of recent decades. The 2,050-word article provided only a shallow analysis of the obesity problem, though. And as he had done in 1998, the *New York Times* article was directed to a tangential issue: whether the low-fat DASH-type or the high-fat Atkins-type diet provided better weight control.

Taubes began his *Times* article by asserting that the typical American diet is a disaster. Then, with a quantum leap he indicted the low-fat high-carbohydrate dietary concept of the American Heart Association and the DASH Research Group. The fault lines in Taubes's thinking became apparent in the initial paragraphs of his piece with his failure to acknowledge that there are different types of carbohydrates and with his inference that, in any case, carbohydrates function identically, points that both Dean Ornish, MD, in an August 2 *New York Times* Op-Ed article[3] and the August–September 2002 *Pritikin Perspective*[4] found necessary to rebut a few days later. Even those who are not educated in such matters understand that there are substantial differences between refined carbohydrates of the donut, cookie, and cake type and the fiber-filled nutrient-packed, straight-from-the-earth carbohydrates of the fruit, vegetable, bean, and whole grain (oats, brown rice, and corn, for instance) type.

First, there is the matter of weight. A refined carbohydrate such as a donut weighs in at 270 calories. Two chocolate cookies contribute 200 calories, a cheddar pretzel, 240 calories.[5] With carbohydrates like those, it doesn't take long to go overboard on calorie consumption.

For the past few decades at least, the focus (prohibition) has been on cholesterol. As long as a dietary item, like a cookie or bagel for instance, is "fat-free," the amount consumed has been considered to not be very important. Not so, of course. In the end, it is calories in (food consumed) versus calories out (energy expended). And calories can quickly add up. What's more, refined carbohydrates lack a proper balance of electrolytes. Cookies, donuts, and the like are positioned near the top of the DASH food pyramid (foods to be avoided).

That's not the case with unrefined carbohydrates—whole foods like fresh fruits, vegetables, grains, and beans. For the most part, unrefined or minimally processed carbohydrates (at the base of the DASH food pyramid) are not dense with calories, not even close. Most vegetables contain 70 to 90 calories per pound. Fresh fruits contain 150 to 425 calories per pound. By contrast, refined carbohydrates like chips, fat-free cookies, and dry cereals add up to a whopping 1,400 to 1,750 calories per pound![6]

The 1997 DASH study established that (1) the substitution of unrefined carbohydrates (fruits, vegetables, and grain products) for refined carbohydrates (sweets, snacks, and the like) lowers blood pressure by 2.8 mm Hg. That switch, while holding fat content constant, added potassium, magnesium, and calcium to the interventional diet. The 1997 study also established that (2) the reduction of total fat (cheese, butter, and the like) and the substitution of low-fat dairy products (skim milk and yogurt) to the enhanced fruit/vegetable diet added calcium and lowered blood pressure by an extra 2.7 mm Hg, for a total reduction of 5.5 mm Hg.

Refined carbohydrates such as cookies and donuts are deficient in potassium, magnesium, and calcium. Fruits and vegetables, on the other hand, contain an abundant amount. What's more, the poster boys for refined carbohydrates—cookies, donuts, muffins, and the like—are high in sodium, often 250 mg or so per serving.[7]

High-Fat Diet Subjected to Clinical Trial

Times readers surely wondered of Gary Taubes's report: What is the medical proof that justifies adherence to the high-fat low-carbohydrate Atkins-type diet? A forthright response would have brought forth the admission that there is none. Actually, the single peer-reviewed study that had investigated the metabolic effects produced by a high-fat low-carbohydrate diet and had been released a few months earlier than the *Times* article was, in a word, frightening. That study was performed at the Osaka City University Medical School in Japan.

One Meal Trial: High-Fat vs. Low-Fat Diet

As reported in the January 2002 issue of *Annals of Internal Medicine*,[8] medical scientists determined that a single high-fat meal reduced blood flow within the heart's coronary arteries. This effect, noted head researcher Takeshi Hozumi, MD, could trigger angina (chest pain caused by insufficient blood flow) in patients with coronary artery disease. Dr. Hozumi measured coronary blood flow in healthy men with an average age of twenty-nine. The determinations were taken both before and after a high-fat meal. Five hours later, the level of small-size fats (triglycerides) within the blood had tripled. And *coronary blood flow had decreased by 18 percent*. The fat molecules had impeded circulatory flow within the coronary arteries.

Next, coronary blood flow was measured in subjects after a low-fat meal. Five hours after the meal, *coronary blood flow had increased rather than decreased*. Triglycerides had risen only slightly.

And what was the Dr. Atkins reply to the Hozumi report? Well, silence. Did his lack of response imply that weight reduction should be the only goal of the high-fat dieter? One would hope not. Blood flow within the coronary arteries is a critical matter. For now, and until additional research is done, Atkins dieters who are experiencing circulatory insufficiency of one type or another should be cautious and seek advice of a physician before continuing further. They might be experiencing a decrease in coronary artery blood flow to a dangerous level.

Next, what happens if a high-fat diet is continued long term? Well, there had not been any specific information until a comparative trial was published in the August 2002 issue of *Preventative Cardiology*.

Twelve Month Trial: 10% vs. 15% vs. 25% vs. 60% Fat Diet

Researchers at the Fleming Heart and Health Institute in Omaha, Nebraska, assigned four different diets to overweight men and women for one year.[9] Patients had to commit to staying on the dietary regimen for a minimum of one year. Average weight for those entering the study was 241 pounds.

The first group followed a diet with 10 percent calories from fat. The diet emphasized complex carbohydrates: fruits, vegetables, and whole grains. The subjects could eat as much as they wanted. Nutritionists who reviewed dietary information supplied by each subject, both during and at the twelve-month termination point for the trial, estimated that on average 1,300 to 1,400 calories had been consumed daily.

The second group was on a calorie-controlled diet with 15 percent calories from fat. This diet also emphasized complex carbohydrates. Those subjects ate 1,500 to 1,600 calories daily.

The third group followed a 20 to 30 percent fat diet and could eat as many calories as they wanted. Nutritionists determined that the subjects in that group consumed 2,000 to 2,200 calories daily.

A fourth group was assigned a high-fat, low-carbohydrate diet similar to the Atkins-type diet. Fat represented 55 to 65 percent of the caloric intake while carbohydrates were reduced to a 10 percent allotment. The diet was not calorie restricted. Nutritionists determined that calories consumed had averaged 1,400 to 1,500 daily.

All four groups were instructed to exercise three to five times weekly. Each bout included fifteen minutes of stretching and thirty minutes of walking.

Weight outcome? Well, those following the *10 percent fat diet showed the greatest weight loss*. In one year, they lost more than 18 percent of their body weight.

Second and third best were those on the 55 to 65 percent fat (Atkins-type) diet and those on the 15 percent fat, calorie-controlled diet. The Atkins dieters lost 13 percent of their body weight. Those following the diet containing 15 percent fat calorie-controlled diet shed 12 percent of their body weight.

The only group that did not lose weight was the 20–30 percent fat group, the one that consumed, far and away, the most calories—2,000 to 2,200 every day. "Clearly, calories count," noted lead investigator Richard M. Fleming, MD. "Regardless of the dietary program used, the key is the same: we must reduce caloric intake to lose weight."

"Weight loss [was] not the only issue that concern[ed] us," Dr. Fleming went on to say. "Popular weight loss programs have appeared that promise weight loss, but they do not address potential health concerns associated with dietary programs." Those concerns were addressed by measurement of several key risk factors for heart disease, including total cholesterol, undesirable LDL cholesterol, desirable HDL cholesterol, and triglycerides.

Risk Factors? After one year, *only one diet showed a worsening of cardiovascular risk factors: the Atkins-type diet*. As Dr. Fleming noted, "The patients on this high-fat diet may have lost weight, but at the price of increased LDL cholesterol, increased triglycerides, increased total cholesterol, [and] decreased HDL cholesterol." Not only did the "risk of heart disease" increase, "but also [did] the risk of stroke, peripheral vascular disease, and blood clot."

Those following the 10 percent and 15 percent fat diets were rewarded not only with weight loss but also with reductions in all the risk factors for heart disease, stroke, and peripheral vascular disease. After one year, total cholesterol for those following the 10 percent fat diet plummeted 38 percent. Those on the 15 percent fat diet decreased total cholesterol by 30 percent. Total cholesterol for the Atkins-type dieters rose 4 percent.

Triglycerides fell 37 percent and 36 percent on the 10 percent and 15 percent fat diets, respectively. On the Atkins-type diet and the 20 to 30 percent fat diets, triglycerides increased.

Concluded Dr. Fleming, "A dietary program may be viewed as helpful as long as it results in weight loss without significant adverse side effects. Our research showed significant adverse side effects with the high-fat diet." "Patients following the high-fat diet showed a worsening of multiple cardiovascular risk factors."

Larry King Live *Interview*

The Taubes *New York Times Magazine* piece stimulated interest in the Atkins diet as never before. Soon, both *Time* (September 2, 2002) and *Newsweek* (January 20, 2003) magazine articles appeared with a text which questioned, as did the *Times* Sunday magazine piece, the validity of the DASH food pyramid. "Is it really O.K.," *Time* mused, "to slather mayonnaise all over salmon and tuna and douse asparagus and lobster with butter while friends look on in envy, as Atkins advocates?" *Time* seemed willing to accept Taubes's dictates:[10] "There are some hints," the *Time* reporter went on to say, "that Atkins may have struck a vein of truth—hints that are intriguing enough to convince some mainstream obesity experts that the approach merits serious consideration."

Newsweek began its article with the declaration:[11] "Something is wrong, if not rotten in the state of New York, the state of California and every state in between. While searching for the right diet, we're consuming ever more calories, growing ever more obese and suffering obscene rates of diabetes, hypertension, and heart disease as a result."

Sandwiched between the *Time* and *Newsweek* articles was a January 6, 2003, CNN *Larry King Live* interview with Dr. Robert

Atkins. Larry King, who has experienced cardiac difficulties of his own, quickly got to some salient points: "The argument against you, was that you were doing all these things without any clinically approved studies."[12] Atkins responded, "Well, I would never do a study because I'm a practicing physician. I mean, all I do is treat people." So, if not from Dr. Atkins, from where does justification for a high-fat diet come? Truth is, from nowhere. After thirty-eight years of medical practice and contact with thousands of patients, Atkins had no published data, nor had there been reports from others to support/justify the high-fat dietary concept.

The Achilles' heel of the Atkins diet has been the concern regarding its effect on blood pressure. The 1997 DASH study showed that a low-fat high-carbohydrate diet reduced blood pressure 5.5 mm Hg in comparison to the standard US diet. A high-fat, low-carbohydrate (Atkins-type) diet would very likely, under the clinical conditions imposed by the DASH researchers, increase the differential another 2 or 3 mm. But Larry King did not bring up that issue. Instead, he went for the other heel, and that is the chemical acidosis which the Atkins diet produces:

> KING: "The *American Journal of Kidney Diseases*, August of 2002,[13] said people on your diet lose large amounts of calcium in the urine, 65 percent higher than normal, 55 percent in maintenance, which possibly could lead to osteoporosis."
> ATKINS: "Well, the calcium loss is very short-term." Then, while finding it difficult to put the words together, he continued, "After two weeks, there is—the calcium level [goes] back to normal. So that's a short-term abnormality."

Apparently, King had been alerted by his medical consultant to inquire about the chemical acidosis produced by the high-fat low-carbohydrate diet. By introducing the results of the *American*

Journal of Kidney Diseases report, King served notice that the Atkins diet has a second fateful flaw. But he failed to follow through and demonstrate that Dr. Atkins had not responded to the question in full.

The 2002 American Journal of Kidney Diseases *Report*

The University of Chicago and University of Texas teams responsible for the study cited by Larry King followed healthy subjects who were placed on an Atkins-type induction diet for two weeks followed by an Atkins-type maintenance diet for four weeks. During the last week of each stage, urine and blood samples were taken for blood acid-base determination, blood electrolyte levels, and urinary electrolyte excretion.

Urine acidity (pH) increased from 6.09, a normal value, to 5.59 during the two-week induction stage. (Note: As acidity increases, the pH value becomes smaller.) During the four-week maintenance stage, urine acidity recovered slightly to a 5.67 pH value—a reading that was still well below the pretest pH determination, nevertheless (fig. 1). Net acid excretion (titratable acidity) doubled during the induction stage and remained near that level during maintenance.

Dietary calcium intake was held constant for each volunteer throughout the dietary trial. Urinary calcium excretion increased significantly, nevertheless, during both the induction and the maintenance phases (fig. 2).

The results of the collaborative study involving the Department of Internal Medicine at the two medical schools was consistent with previous reports showing that high-protein diets deliver an exaggerated acid load. The authors emphasized that the change in urine acidity and the increased calcium excretion would enhance the propensity for kidney stone formation. The implication of the increased calcium excretion on bone metabolism was also apparent.

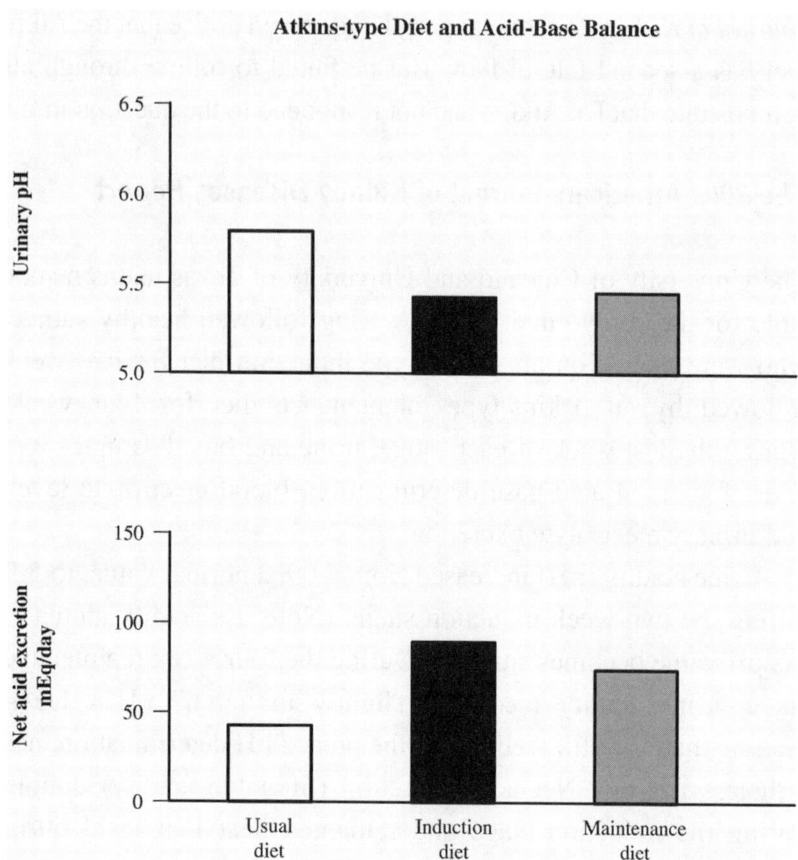

Fig. 1. Effect of Atkins-type diet on acid-base balance. Urinary pH decreased significantly during induction and remained so during the maintenance phase. Net acid excretion (titratable acidity and ammonium values minus the calculated urinary bicarbonate) increased almost twofold. (Reproduced with permission from Reddy, ST et al. *American Journal of Kidney Diseases* 2002;**40**:265–274)

The authors considered osteoporosis to be a distinct risk for those who continue an Atkins-type diet for an extended period of time.

Dr. Atkins responded to Larry King by agreeing that calcium is lost from the body during the two-week period of induction, but he was either unaware that the *American Journal of Kidney Diseases* report also showed that calcium continues to be lost during the

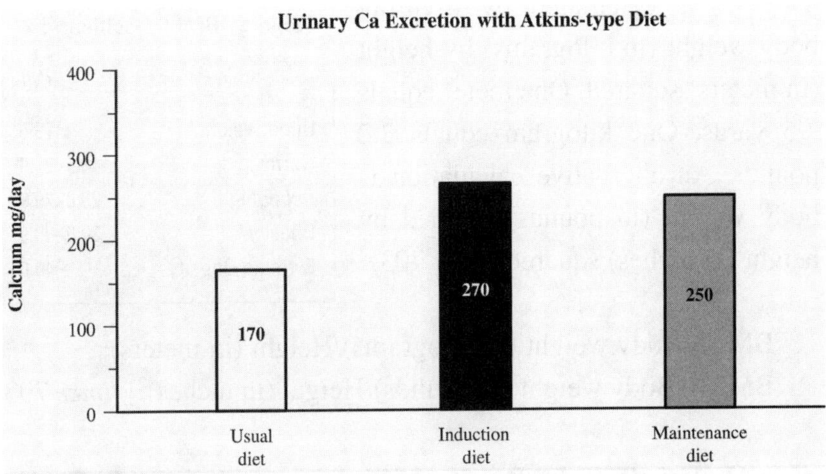

Fig. 2. Effect of Atkins-type diet on urinary excretion of calcium. Urinary calcium increased substantially following adherence to Atkins diet. ($p < 0.001$ for induction diet and < 0.01 for maintenance diet). (Reprinted with permission from the *American Journal of Kidney Diseases*)

maintenance phase or was unwilling to accept that portion of their findings. The long-term risk to bone health of the Atkins diet is surely an issue that will be raised again and again.[14]

OBESITY

Gary Taubes's *New York Times Magazine* piece specifically indicted the low-fat high-carbohydrate diet for the obesity epidemic of the past thirty years. For some time now, health specialists have classified obesity by Body Mass Index (BMI), a measurement that takes into account both weight and height[15] (table 1). A man or woman who is five feet five and weighs 132 pounds has a BMI of 22, which is considered normal. A BMI of 25 to 30 falls into the overweight category. A BMI over 30 is considered obese.

BMI is calculated by dividing body weight (in kilograms) by height (in meters) squared. One meter equals .95 yards. One kilogram equals 2.2 pounds. An alternative calculation is body weight (in pounds) divided by height (in inches) squared *times* 703.

Table 1. BMI Classification

	BMI
Underweight	< 18.5
Normal	18.5–24.9
Overweight	25.0–29.9
Obesity	30.0–39.9
Extreme Obesity	≥ 40.0

BMI = Body weight (in kilograms)/Height (in meters)^2
BMI = [Body weight (in pounds)/Height (in inches)^2] *times* 703

Body Mass Index Table

	19	20	21	22	23	24	25	26	27	28	29	30	31	32	33	34	35
Height (inches)	Body Weight (pounds)																
58	91	96	100	105	110	115	119	124	129	134	138	143	148	153	158	162	167
59	94	99	104	109	114	119	124	128	133	138	143	148	153	158	163	168	173
60	97	102	107	112	118	123	128	133	138	143	148	153	158	163	168	174	179
61	100	106	111	116	122	127	132	137	143	148	153	158	164	169	174	180	185
62	104	109	115	120	126	131	136	142	147	153	158	164	169	175	180	186	191
63	107	113	118	124	130	135	141	146	152	158	163	169	175	180	186	191	197
64	110	116	122	128	134	140	145	151	157	163	169	174	180	186	192	197	204
65	114	120	126	132	138	144	150	156	162	168	174	180	186	192	198	204	210
66	118	124	130	136	142	148	155	161	167	173	179	186	192	198	204	210	216
67	121	127	134	140	146	153	159	166	172	178	185	191	198	204	211	217	223
68	125	131	138	144	151	158	164	171	177	184	190	197	203	210	216	223	230
69	128	135	142	149	155	162	169	176	182	189	196	203	209	216	223	230	236
70	132	139	146	153	160	167	174	181	188	195	202	209	216	222	229	236	243
71	136	143	150	157	165	172	179	186	193	200	208	215	222	229	236	243	250
72	140	147	154	162	169	177	184	191	199	206	213	221	228	235	242	250	258
73	144	151	159	166	174	182	189	197	204	212	219	227	235	242	250	257	265
74	148	155	163	171	179	186	194	202	210	218	225	233	241	249	256	264	272
75	152	160	168	176	184	192	200	208	216	224	232	240	248	256	264	272	279
76	156	164	172	180	189	197	205	213	221	230	238	246	254	263	271	279	287

Fig. 3A. Height, in inches, is read in the left-hand column. Then, slide over to body weight. The corresponding number above is the Body Mass Index. BMI 19–35, left side (Fig. 3A). BMI 36–54, right side (Fig. 3B).

If the math is painful, one can find instant calculators online (try nhlbisupport.com). For the physician, tables have been devised to permit rapid determination of BMI (figs. 3A and 3B).

If our example subject gains 50 pounds, the BMI reaches 30, and she is considered obese. According to the most recent National Health and Examination Survey (NHANES 2002),[16] 34 percent of US adults (48 million) are overweight (BMI 25–29.9) and an additional 31 percent (44 million) are obese (BMI above 30). Of the latter group, 6 million are considered extremely obese (BMI ≥ 40); they weigh about 100 pounds more than they should.

The statistical breakdown for the 92 million US overweight and obese individuals by age, sex, and racial/ethnic group is shown in table 2.

Body Mass Index Table

Height (inches)	36	37	38	39	40	41	42	43	44	45	46	47	48	49	50	51	52	53	54
	Body Weight (pounds)																		
58	172	177	181	186	191	196	201	205	210	215	220	224	229	234	239	244	248	253	258
59	178	183	188	193	198	203	208	212	217	222	227	232	237	242	247	252	257	262	267
60	184	189	194	199	204	209	215	220	225	230	235	240	245	250	255	261	266	271	276
61	190	195	201	206	211	217	222	227	232	238	243	248	254	259	264	269	275	280	285
62	196	202	207	213	218	224	229	235	240	246	251	256	262	267	273	278	284	289	295
63	203	208	214	220	225	231	237	242	248	254	259	265	270	278	282	287	293	299	304
64	209	215	221	227	232	238	244	250	256	262	267	273	279	285	291	296	302	308	314
65	216	222	228	234	240	246	252	258	264	270	276	282	288	294	300	306	312	318	324
66	223	229	235	241	247	253	260	266	272	278	284	291	297	303	309	315	322	328	334
67	230	236	242	249	255	261	268	274	280	287	293	299	306	312	319	325	331	338	344
68	236	243	249	256	262	269	276	282	289	295	302	308	315	322	328	335	341	348	354
69	243	250	257	263	270	277	284	291	297	304	311	318	324	331	338	345	351	358	365
70	250	257	264	271	278	285	292	299	306	313	320	327	334	341	348	355	362	369	376
71	257	265	272	279	286	293	301	308	315	322	329	338	343	351	358	365	372	379	386
72	265	272	279	287	294	302	309	316	324	331	338	346	353	361	368	375	383	390	397
73	272	280	288	295	302	310	318	325	333	340	348	355	363	371	378	386	393	401	408
74	280	287	295	303	311	319	326	334	342	350	358	365	373	381	389	396	404	412	420
75	287	295	303	311	319	327	335	343	351	359	367	375	383	391	399	407	415	423	431
76	295	304	312	320	328	336	344	353	361	369	377	385	394	402	410	418	426	435	443

Fig. 3B.

Table 2. Overweight and Obese by Age, Sex, and Racial/Ethnic Group: United States, 1999–2000

		Incidence (%) Overweight and Obese BMI ≥ 25		
Sex	*Age*	*White*	*Black*	*Hispanic*
Men	≤ 20	67	61	75
	20–39	61	53	68
	40–59	70	64	79
	≥ 60	74	69	80
Women	≤ 20	57	57	77
	20–39	49	49	71
	40–59	61	61	82
	≥ 60	66	66	82

(Modified with permission from Flegal, KM *Journal of the American Medical Association* 2002;**288**:1723–1727)

The age-adjusted prevalence trend of obesity and extreme obesity from 1960 to 2002 is shown in figure 4. The incidence of obesity was relatively constant from 1960 to 1980, only to increase to significantly higher levels since then.

The American Heart Association issued its initial low-fat, sodium-restricted dietary recommendations in 1957[17] when heart disease was becoming more prevalent. That position was reinforced in 1961, in 1965,[18] and on several subsequent occasions.[19] Gary Taubes pointed out in the *Times* piece that obesity became a serious public health problem during the same period that the American Heart Association actively pursued dietary recommendations. Guilt by association, he contends. Could he be right? Hardly.

Medical researchers do predict that *obesity will be the major chronic health problem of the Western world throughout the twenty-first century.*[20] Obesity has already reached epidemic proportions in several

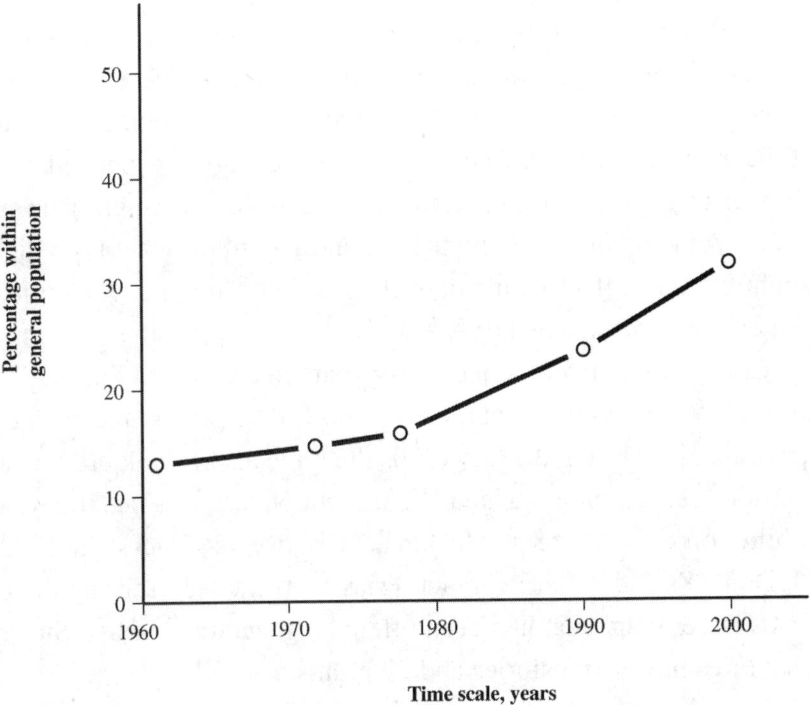

Fig. 4. Trend in prevalence of obesity for US adults 20–74 years, 1960–2000. (Data extracted with permission from Flegal, KM et al *Journal of the American Medical Association* 2002;**288**:1723–1727)

nations. The rise in incidence has a number of explanations, surely, but genetics is not one of them. A change in gene pool cannot account for a radical increase in prevalence in just one or two generations.

What has changed is our way of eating and living. In simple terms, when people eat more and move less, they get fat. Unfortunately, energy expenditure has not been calculated historically, but several trends are evident. Fewer people walk or bike than ever before. The automobile has become the means of locomotion. And mechanization has alleviated toil on the farm, in the workplace, and in the office. What's more, fewer people engage in leisure-time physical activity. In 1995, 28.8 percent of those polled by the Centers for Disease Control reported no leisure-time physical activity.[21] More and more time is spent in the comfort of one's home, in front of the television set or the computer. If less energy is expended, the number of calories consumed must be decreased if weight gain is to be avoided. Numerous myths abound regarding what type diet might be most effective in controlling weight. In the end, calories and only calories make a difference.

Consider that over the past forty years in the United States, per capita consumption of carbonated soft drinks has more than quadrupled.[22] During the late 1950s the typical soft drink order at a fast-food restaurant contained about eight ounces of soda; today, a "child" order of Coke at McDonald's is twelve ounces. In 1972 McDonald's added Large French Fries to its menu; a serving three times larger than what had been offered a generation earlier. Super Size Fries have 610 calories and 29 grams of fat.[23]

To sell their products in an economy of abundant choices, food companies employ aggressive marketing strategies. Manufacturers introduce thousands of new food and beverage products into the market every year. Food and food service companies spend more than $11 billion annually on direct media advertising. As a result, the calories provided by the US food supply have increased from 3,300 per capita in 1970 to 3,800 in the late 1990s, a statistic that surely provides the explanation for the rise of obesity among Americans over the same time period.

Although general consensus holds that food portions have been increasing in size and that the increase is one factor contributing to the obesity epidemic in the United States, no data has been available until recently to document that trend. In January 2003 the US Department of Agriculture and the Food and Drug Administration jointly published data showing that most foods, with one or two exceptions, are available in larger portions than they were in the 1970s.[24] The data from three nationally representative surveys comprising individuals age two and older were employed. Three food sources were compiled: (1) eaten at home, which presently represents 65 percent of total calories consumed, (2) served at fast-food outlets, and (3) served at traditional restaurants.

The food categories analyzed were salty snacks, desserts, french fries, hamburgers, cheeseburgers, pizza, and Mexican food. Overall portion sizes for these foods, other than pizza, increased during the interval of study (1977–1996). The incremental change was substantial and enough to cause, if the portion was completely consumed, a substantial increase in weight per year (fig. 5).

For most of the selected foods, fast-food outlets served the largest portions, the investigators found. That might relate to "value adding" pricing practices whereby fast-food outlets add larger portions for either little or no cost increase. During the twenty-year interval that was studied, the researchers found that portion size also increased for food consumed at home while traditional restaurants had made little change in size.

The obesity epidemic that began in the United States during the 1970s and now includes many other nations has spread, surely, with fast food as one of its vectors. Between 1984 and 1993, the number of fast-food restaurants in Great Britain doubled—and so did the obesity rate among adults.[25] Overweight people were once a rarity in Japan. The nation's traditional diet of rice, fish, vegetables, and soy products has been deemed one of the healthiest in the world. In recent years the Japanese have been abandoning that diet. The arrival of McDonald's in 1971 accelerated the shift in eating habits. During the 1980s, the sale of fast food in Japan more than doubled, and obesity among children increased, too.[26]

What is particularly, perhaps uniquely, challenging about obe-

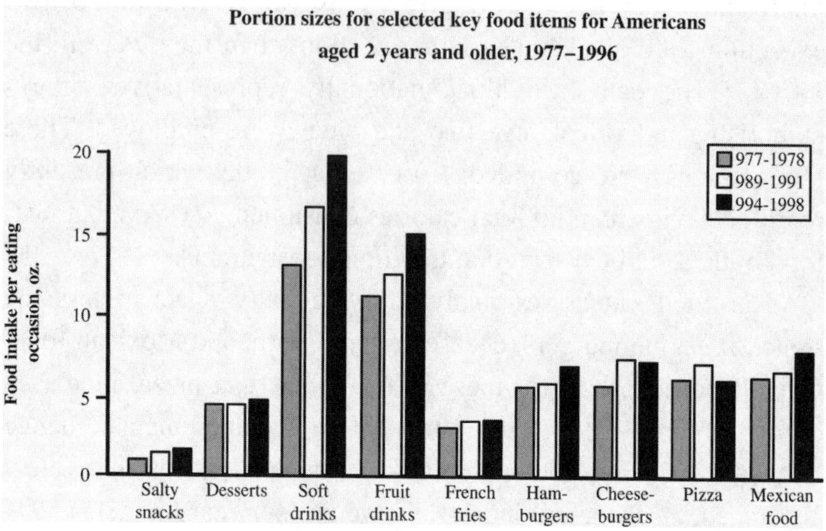

Fig. 5. Portion sizes for selected key food items for Americans aged two years and older, 1977–1996. (Reproduced with permission from Nielson, SJ *Journal of the American Medical Association* 2003;**289**:449–453)

sity is that everyone, professionals and nonprofessionals alike, has an opinion about the causes and remedies for the condition. Regrettably, these are often just opinions based on selective evidence for their derivation. The 1998 National Institutes of Health (NIH) publication "Clinical Guidelines on the Identification, Evaluation, and Treatment of Overweight and Obesity in Adults: The Evidence Report"[27] has been a major breakthrough. It serves as an authoritative framework for the facilitation of communication and the implementation of treatment.

Clinicians have rigorously investigated different diet comparatives that could be effective in enhancing weight loss, including very-low-fat, low-fat, high-fiber, low-carbohydrate, and high-protein weight-reducing meal plans. The overriding conclusions from those studies are that calorie intake is the major determinant for weight loss and that variation in fat, protein, and carbohydrates do not have a significant impact on weight. Thus, diet composition is primarily important in terms of health maintenance and in disease prevention. Weight loss requires a calorie deficit. And the general consensus is that cake, cookies, butter, cheese, and the like are where the restriction begins.

Obesity requires the attention of all health professionals. The epidemic extends far beyond emotional pain and low self-esteem. The Centers for Disease Control and Prevention estimates that 280,000 Americans die every year as a direct result of being overweight. Obesity has been linked to heart disease, colon cancer, breast cancer, respiratory insufficiency (fig. 6), diabetes, arthritis (the weight-bearing joints—hip, knee, and ankle—in particular), high blood pressure, infertility, and stroke.[28]

Researchers have found, furthermore, that individuals who are overweight/obese throughout adulthood are more likely to experience brain atrophy (shrinkage) as they become older. In one study of 290 Swedish women,[29] those who were overweight during a twenty-four-year observation period were significantly more likely to experience a decrease in brain size, as determined by MRI (x-ray).

The researchers found that for every one-point gain in BMI, the risk of brain shrinkage increased by 13 to 16 percent!

The authors explained that overweight people are more likely to have high blood pressure, hypercholesterolemia (elevated blood cholesterol level), and diabetes—conditions that contribute to blood vessel damage within the brain. They concluded that an abnormally elevated BMI should be considered a risk factor for the development of senility, dementia, and Alzheimer's disease.

Finally, an abnormally elevated BMI in adulthood is associated, not surprisingly, with a decreases in life expectancy and an increased likelihood of early mortality[30] (fig. 7). These decreases are similar to those seen with smoking. Obesity in adulthood is a

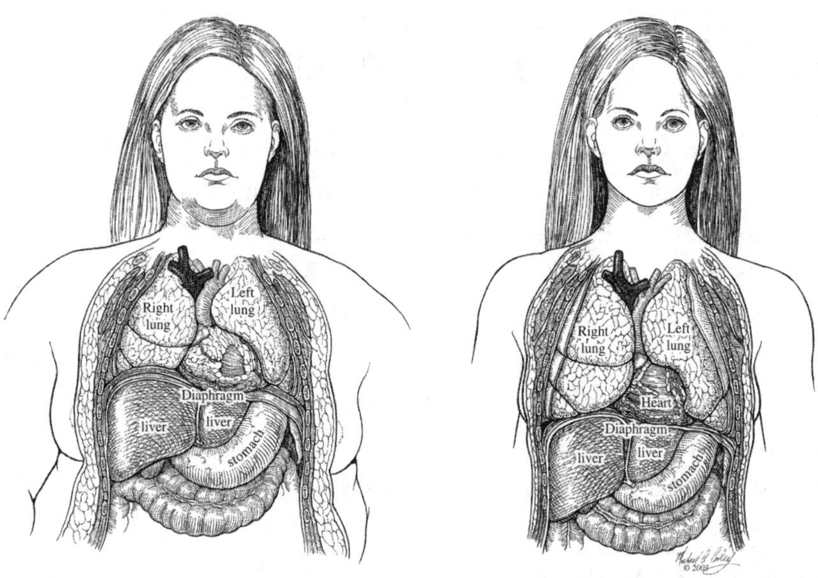

Fig. 6. The respiratory insufficiency that obese people experience is to no small measure the result of lung compression. A protuberant abdomen produces upward pressure on the diaphragm, the flat muscle that supports the lungs and separates the abdomen from the chest cavity (above, on left). The compression on the lungs reduces oxygen saturation of the circulatory system with the result that a frequent complaint for severely overweight individuals is shortness of breath and easy fatigability.

With loss of weight (above, on right), fat encasing the heart diminishes and the contractile force of the ventricle improves. Weight loss allows the lungs to expand as the diaphragm and abdominal organs descend. With the extension of the respiratory excursions, blood oxygenation improves promptly to the normal range. (See *Bulletin of the Walter Kempner Foundation* 1972, vol. 4, no. 1)

powerful predictor of death at older ages. The data indicate that obesity is far worse than just a cosmetic problem.

Gary Taubes concluded his piece with a confession, of sorts. He, like so many others, has a tendency for corpulence. He implied that an Atkins-type diet would be the next step for him. He will lose weight if restraint is demonstrated, but he will not be doing his cho-

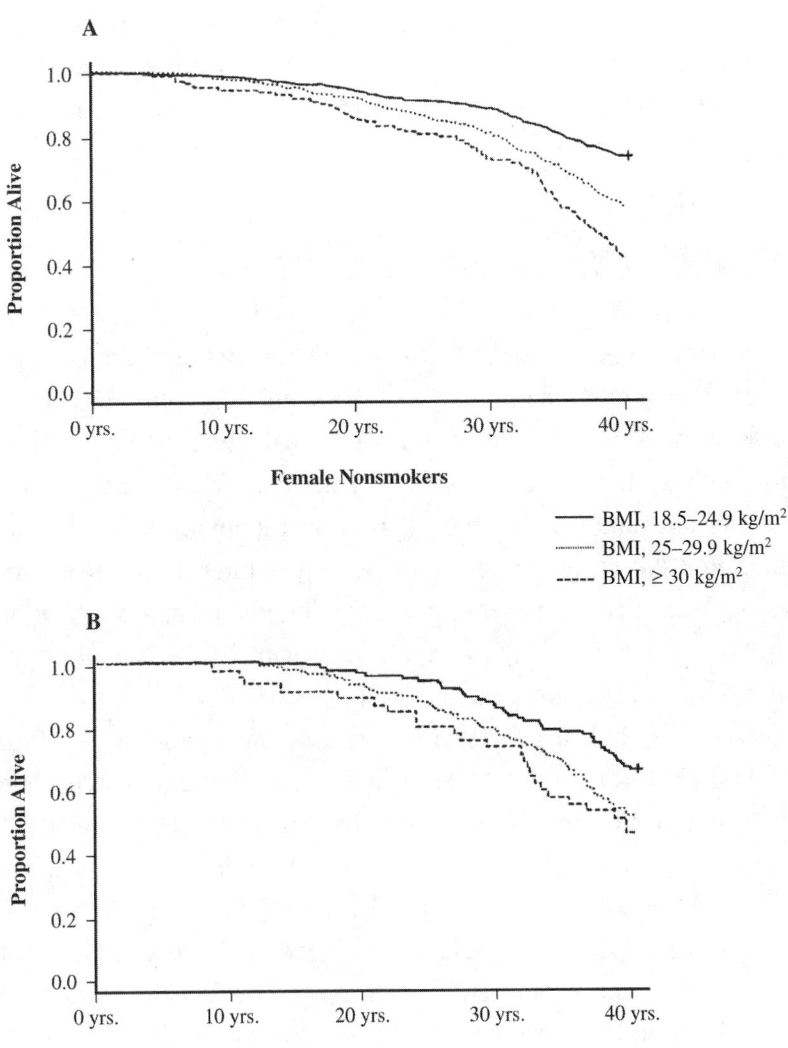

Fig. 7. Survival estimate for body mass index. Obesity in adulthood at age forty (0 years on the horizontal axis) and its future consequences for life expectancy (over the next four decades). Nonsmokers. Female above. Male below. (Reproduced with permission from Peter, A et al *Annals of Internal Medicine* 2003;**138**:24–31)

lesterol count a favor, as the Fleming Heart and Health Institute determined. And because the electrolyte intake for the Atkins-type diet is far removed from the DASH ideal, he will not be doing his blood pressure or his calcium metabolism a favor, either.

SPINNING A YARN—SETTING THE BAR

As Barbara Rolls, an obesity expert at Pennsylvania State University, explained in *Nutrition Action*,[31] a few months following publication of the Taubes "What If It's All Been a Big Fat Lie?" article, "He [Taubes] knows how to spin a yarn. What frightens me is that he picks and chooses his facts." Bonnie Liebman, author of the *Nutrition Action* article, reported that Taubes interviewed Rolls for six hours and that Rolls sent him a huge bundle of papers. "But he didn't quote a word of it," Rolls told Liebman. "If the facts don't fit with his yarn, he ignores them."

John Farquhar, a professor emeritus of medicine at Stanford University's Center for Research in Disease Prevention who had been quoted in the Taubes *New York Times* piece, stated to Liebman, "He [Taubes] took this weird little idea and blew it up, and people believed him." "What a disaster," he went on to say.

Others interviewed by Liebman agreed. "It's silly to say that carbohydrates cause obesity," said George Blackburn of Harvard Medical School. "We're overweight because we overeat calories."

The response of Gerald Reaven of Stanford University was particularly telling. His comments had appeared in the Taubes article. "My quote was correct," he told Liebman, "but the context suggested that I support eating saturated fat." He went on to say, "I was horrified," and "The article was terribly misleading."

Liebman also noted that the *Washington Post* had asked Taubes why he made no mention of a review of nearly fifty studies on weight loss in the National Heart, Lung, and Blood Institute's 1998 Clinical Guidelines on treating obesity. The panel of experts had been chaired by Columbia University's F. X. Pi-Sunyer, who has served as president of both the American Society of Clinical Nutrition and the American Diabetes Association.

"Anything that Pi-Sunyer is involved with, I don't take seriously," said Taubes to the *Post* reporter. "He doesn't strike me as a scientist."[32] Taubes did not explain, incidentally, how he, a reporter, was qualified to question the expertise of Pi-Sunyer, a respected scientist. Liebman ended her analysis of the Taubes piece with this paragraph:

> Readers expect the [*New York*] *Times* [*Magazine*] to run articles that are honestly reported and written. . . . If Taubes had written a news article for the front page of the *Times*, comments like those would have ended his career. But when it comes to reporting about diet, the bar is set lower. Surely, the public deserves better.

Take notice, Salt Institute. Backlash from the Taubes *New York Times* piece could signal a new attitude about nutritional reporting. What is sorely needed are facts, not prejudices. The public is certain to demand that the bar be raised.

NOTES

1. Taubes, G. What if it's all been a big fat lie? *New York Times Magazine*. July 2, 2002.

2. Taubes, G. The (political) science of salt. *Science* 1998;**281**:898–907.

3. Ornish, D. A diet rich in partial truths. *New York Times*. July 13, 2002.

4. Novick, J. Pritikin doctors challenge *New York Times Magazine* article: what if it's all been a big fat lie? Pritikin *Perspective*. Vol. 2, No. 8:1–3.

5. Netzer, CT. *The Complete Book of Food Counts*. New York: Dell Publishing, 1994.

6. Ibid.

7. Ibid.

8. Hozumi, T. et al High-fat meals reduce coronary blood flow. *Annals of Internal Medicine* 2002;**136**:523–528.

9. Fleming, RN. The effect of high-, moderate-, and low-fat diets on weight loss and cardiovascular disease risk factors. *Preventative Cardiology* (Summer 2002):110–118.

10. Nash, JM. Cracking the fat riddle. *Time* September 2, 2002, pp. 45–55.

11. Cowley, G. A better way to eat. *Newsweek* January 20, 2003, http://www.msnbc.com/news/857556.

12. King, L. Interview with Robert Atkins, http://www.cnn.com/TRANSCRIPTS.

13. Reddy, ST. Effect of low-carbohydrate high-protein diets on acid-base balance, stone-forming propensity, and calcium metabolism. *American Journal of Kidney Disease* 2002;**40**:265–274.

14. Indeed, Dr. Atkins was next pressured about the *American Journal of Kidney Diseases* report during an April 2003 interview with a *Journal of the American Medical Association* editor. For the complete transcript see Stephenson, J. Low-carb, low-fat diet gurus face off. *JAMA* 2003;**289**:1767–1775.

> *JAMA*: Many have expressed concerns about the long-term safety of a low-carbohydrate diet, such as the effects of calcium loss on bone, or whether the relatively high protein content might be a problem for people who have a propensity to form kidney stones.
>
> DR. ATKINS: We've never seen it. But nobody's done a study on long-term use of any diet.

Dr. Atkins was accompanied to the interview session by Colette Heimowitz, MS, director of education and research at Atkins Health & Medical Information Services. She added to Dr. Atkins's response as follows:

MEIMOWITZ: Concerns come from the initial water loss in the first few days when there's a slight shift in pH and a slight loss of electrolytes, but that quickly returns to baseline. That's why taking a multivitamin and potassium citrate and drinking adequate water is very important in the induction phase, when about 35% of calories are from protein, to counteract the side effects of the initial weight loss.

Heimowitz indicated that the urinary pH and the loss of calcium return to baseline. But that was not the findings of the researchers who authored the *American Journal of Kidney Diseases* report. Dr. Atkins's response to the *JAMA* questioning can only be regarded as evasive. Certainly, he did not indicate that he had begun monitoring acid-base balance and urine calcium loss for his patients.

15. Mastbaum, LI and Gumbiner, B. Medical assessment and treatment of the obese patient. In: *Obesity*. Gumbiner, B. (ed.). East Peoria, IL: Versa Press, 2001, pp. 102–130.

16. Flegal, KM et al. Prevalence and trends of obesity among US adults, 1999–2000. *JAMA* 2002;**288**:1723–1739.

17. Page, IH et al. Atherosclerosis and the fat content of the diet. *JAMA* 1957;**164:**2048–2051.

18. Report by the Central Committee for Medical and Community Program for the American Heart Association. Dietary fat and its relation to heart attacks and strokes. *Circulation* 1961;**23**:133–136.

American Heart Association. *Diet and Heart Disease*. New York: American Heart Association, 1965.

19. American Heart Association. *Diet and Heart Disease*. New York: American Heart Association, 1968.

American Heart Association. *Diet and Coronary Heart Disease*. New York: American Heart Association, 1973.

American Heart Association. Diet and coronary heart disease: a statement for physicians and other health professionals. *Circulation* 1978;**54**:762A–766A.

American Heart Association. Dietary guidelines for healthy American adults: a statement for physicians and health professionals by the Nutrition Committee. *Circulation* 1986;**74**:1465A–1468A.

American Heart Association. Dietary guidelines for healthy American adults: a statement for physicians and health professionals by the Nutrition Committee. *Circulation* 1988;**7**:721A–724A.

American Heart Association. The healthy American diet. *Circulation* 1991;**82**:1079.

US Dietary Guideline Committee, US Department of Agriculture, US Department of Health and Human Services. Nutrition and your health: dietary guidelines for Americans. *Home & Garden Bulletin*. 4th ed. 1995:232.

American Heart Association. Dietary guidelines for healthy American adults: a statement for health professionals from the Nutrition Committee. *Circulation* 1996;**94**:1795–1800.

American Heart Association. ADA dietary guidelines revision 2000. *Circulation* 2000;**102**:2284–2299.

20. Pi-Sunyer, FX et al. Therapeutic controversy: obesity—a modern-day epidemic. *Journal of Clinical Endocrinology and Metabolism* 1999;**84**:3–11.

21. Williamson, D et al. Recreational physical activity and ten-year weight change in a US national cohort. *International Journal of Obesity* 1993;**17**:279–284.

22. Schlosser, E. *Fast Food Nation*. New York: HarperCollins, 2002, p. 241.

23. Ibid., p. 241.

24. Nelson, SJ. Patterns and trends in food portion sizes. *JAMA* 1997–1998;**289**:450–453.

25. Schlosser, E. *Fast Food Nation*. New York: HarperCollins, 2002, p. 242.

26. Ibid.

27. NHLBI Obesity Education Expert Panel. *Clinical Guidelines on the Identification, Evaluation, and Treatment of Overweight and Obesity in Adults: The Evidence Report.* Bethesda, MD: National Institute of Health, National Heart, Lung, and Blood Institute. NIH Publication 98-4083, 1998.

28. Colovitz, GA. Epidemiology of obesity. In: *Obesity.* Gumbiner, B (ed.). East Peoria, IL: Versa Press, 2001, pp. 1–22.

29. Gustafson, D et al. A 24-year follow-up of body mass index and cerebral atrophy. *Neurology* 2004;**63**:1876–1881.

30. Peters, A et al. Obesity in adulthood and its consequences for life expectancy: life-table analysis. *Annals of Internal Medicine* 2003;**138**:24–32.

Fontaine, KR. Years of life lost to obesity. *JAMA* 2003;**289**:187–193.

Flegal, KM et al. Excess deaths associated with underweight, overweight, and obesity. *JAMA* 2005;**293**:1861–1867.

31. Liebman, B. The truth about the Atkins Diet. *Nutrition Action* 2002;**29**:1–7.

32. According to Dr. F. X. Pi-Sunyer's biographical sketch, he obtained a bachelor of arts from Oberlin College, a medical degree from Columbia University College of Physicians and Surgeons, and a master of public health degree from Harvard University. His research interests are in the hormonal control of carbohydrate metabolism, diabetes mellitus, obesity, and food-intake regulation. He has published 110 original scientific papers; more than 80 nonexperimental articles, chapters, or reviews; and 2 books. Dr. Pi-Sunyer is a past president of the American Diabetes Association, of the American Society for Clinical Nutrition, and of the North American Association for the Study of Obesity. He has been honored as a Fellow of the Fogarty International Center of the National Institutes of Health. He serves on the NIDDK Task Force for the Prevention and Treatment of Obesity and has been a member of numerous NIH study sections and review groups. He is presently chairman of the National Heart and Lung Institute Task Force on the Treatment of Obesity. He is a member of the New York State Health Research Council. He is editor-in-chief of *Obesity Research* and is on the editorial board of the *International Journal of Obesity.*

CHAPTER 11

EVENTS OF APRIL/MAY 2003

In April 2003 Robert C. Atkins died suddenly. A month later two studies appeared in the *New England Journal of Medicine*[1] comparing the weight-reduction potential of high-fat and low-fat diets. Some news sources felt that the results of the *NEJM* reports had validated Atkins's dietary concepts at long last. But researchers who analyzed the data felt otherwise. There was nothing in either report that lent support for the high-fat dietary concept.

ROBERT C. ATKINS, RIP (10/17/30–4/17/03)

On April 8, 2003, Robert Atkins fell while walking to his Manhattan office and was rushed to nearby New York Weill-Cornell Medical Center where he died nine days later.[2]

Atkins was born in Columbus, Ohio. After completion of premedical studies at the University of Michigan, he received a medical degree from Cornell University Medical School in 1955. Residency training was in internal medicine at hospitals affiliated with the University of Rochester and Columbia University. He commenced his medical practice on Manhattan's Upper East Side in 1959.

Atkins liked to tell the story of the lack of self-esteem he endured as his weight increased to 193 pounds by age thirty-three. It was at that point he read about and became interested in a no-carbohydrate dietary regimen pioneered by Dr. Alfred W. Pennington. In desperation Atkins applied that concept to himself, and in just a few weeks twenty pounds were shed. A little later he was hired by the American Telephone and Telegraph company to provide weight counseling. Of the sixty-five AT&T employees he monitored with a weight problem, sixty-four were able to get down to their ideal weight.

Word about Atkins's dietary regimen spread especially after he appeared on the *Tonight* television program in 1965 with Buddy Hackett, an entertainment celebrity. Newspapers described Atkins's dietary concept that became known as the *Vogue diet* after the magazine which published it in 1970. He advised dieters to choose "bacon and eggs over fruit salad" and "truly luxurious foods without limitation." He promised that "lobster dripping with butter," "steak with béarnaise," and "bacon cheeseburgers" were better for weight loss than a bran muffin.

Atkins's practice flourished. By 1972 his first book, *Dr. Atkins' Diet Revolution*, was released. In 1974 the American Medical Association labeled the diet as "potentially dangerous," "naïve," and "biochemically incorrect." Despite the professional opposition Atkins's books sold fifteen million copies over the next thirty years as millions tried his high-fat high-protein dietary concept. His regimen reached peak popularity in the 1990s with the publication of *Dr. Atkins' New Diet Revolution*, which, alone, sold ten million copies worldwide and spent five years on the *New York Times* best-seller list.

Alternative Medicine

Atkins's clinical practice was not limited to weight counseling. Increasingly, he turned to alternative types of therapy for the medical problems of his patients. In his book *Dr. Atkins' Health Revolution* and during interviews, he maintained that ozone gas, a form of oxygen, could kill cancer cells and HIV, the virus that causes AIDS.

Molecules of ordinary oxygen are made of two oxygen atoms joined tightly together. Ozone molecules have a third oxygen atom loosely attached to the other two. The third atom can easily separate from the molecule and combine with other substances. As a result, ozone is a chemically active gas.

Atkins claimed that he had treated more than one thousand patients with ozone therapy. He never published results of such therapy. In fact, he never published a clinical report of any type.

Atkins denounced, in his book, the American Cancer Society, the leading cancer hospitals, the National Cancer Institute, and the Federal Drug Administration for not following his lead in employing ozone for cancer therapy. But they had given ozone a fair review. He remarked, nevertheless, that those institutions are dominated by the pharmaceutical industry, which profits so incredibly much from the industry-made obsession with chemotherapy.

He disparaged chemotherapy, which despite its unpleasant side effects has extended the life expectancy of innumerable cancer patients. Lance Armstrong, who at one time was ravaged by metastatic testicular cancer, is just one notable example of the efficacy of such treatment.[3] Atkins was proud to say that his pathway was that of alternative medicine. To many he was thought of as a trailblazer, and as a result he attracted many frustrated and desperate patients.

He prescribed a wide array of pharmaceutical products—vitamins, antioxidants, herbs, mineral concoctions, enzymes, and supplements of all types—which were packaged with an "Atkins Certified" label and sold through pharmaceutical outlets associated with the Atkins Institute, as his practice was so designated. His books listed a complex array of substances to take not only for general health maintenance but also for sleep, pain, acute infection, high blood pressure, heart disease, arthritis, fatigue, osteoporosis, and on and on. The pharmaceutical outlet, Atkins Nutritionals, which he established to sell diet foods and supplements, consistently accounted for more than $100 million in revenue each year. The products offered through his online sales outlet, Atkinsstore.com, numbered several hundred.

Many of his patients with blood vessel and heart disease received a particular type of alternative therapy, chelation, which knowledgeable researchers summarily dismiss as unorthodox and unproven. By that technique a medication was infused into the patient by intravenous drip, in Atkins's office, and as it passes out of the body, unwanted toxins, according to the description in Atkins's book, are carried away.

Chelation has never been shown in peer-reviewed medical studies to reverse heart disease or any other problem. Its use has been rejected by the American Medical Association and other health agencies. That objection did not bother Atkins. Thousands of patients were subjected to chelation even though scientific proof of efficacy remained elusive.

New York Times

Following publication of Gary Taubes's "What If It's All Been a Big Fat Lie?" piece in the July 2001 *New York Times Magazine*, Atkins's *Dr. Atkins New Diet Revolution* rose four notches on the best-seller list and his *Atkins for Life* zoomed from number 183 to number 5.

Cardiomyopathy

On April 18, 2002, Atkins experienced cardiac arrest while eating breakfast at a restaurant near his medical office. Dining with him was a medical associate who revived Atkins and transported him to nearby Columbia Presbyterian Hospital. Heart attack was ruled out and following a week of treatment and observation, Atkins was discharged.

A press release was provided by the Atkins organization on April 25. It was disclosed that Atkins had developed a heart problem two years earlier and that he had been under the care of Patrick Fratellone, MD, a cardiologist, since that time. The heart difficulty was labeled cardiomyopathy, which means that the heart muscle has become dilated and weakened. Contractile force becomes diminished. During the prior evaluation (in 2000), the coronary arteries were found to have a "normal" angiographic configuration. More specific details were not forthcoming. Normal could have referred to the comparative appearance with that of other sixty-five- to seventy-year-old men, many of whom are found to exhibit, on angiographic evaluation, partial blockage of one or more coronary arteries. Or, perhaps, normal could have meant that there was no evidence of cholesterol deposition whatsoever, which would be the finding for a twenty-year-old.

In the news release the Atkins organization explained that "cardiopathy is a non-coronary condition" which in no way "is related to diet." But should they have been so confident? Consider that the Hozumi trial, referred to in chapter 10, found that a high-fat diet actually reduces blood flow to the heart muscle irrespective of the presence/absence of cholesterol deposition within the coronary arteries. Atkins was a forty-year guinea pig for the high-fat high-protein dietary concept. Such a regimen could have caused injury to the muscle fibers of the heart despite the fact that a significant degree of cholesterol deposition, according to the coronary angiogram of two years earlier, had not formed within the coronary arteries.

A Fall to the Sidewalk

In April 2003, the Atkins Foundation did not provide a news release about Atkins's death. The newspaper account said that Atkins fell and struck his head. One can surmise that bleeding within the brain became apparent following admission to the hospital since, according to the news accounts, an operative procedure, drainage of the blood and decompression of the brain, was done during the period of hospital confinement.

Atkins's physicians were confronted with two explanations for the intracranial bleeding. First, his head could have struck the sidewalk violently and the bleeding could have developed as a result of traumatic rupture of a blood vessel. Second, Atkins could have sustained, while walking down the sidewalk, the spontaneous rupture of a blood vessel within his brain. Information was not forthcoming regarding the status of Dr. Atkins's blood pressure. An elevated blood pressure would be a predisposing risk factor for the latter.

With traumatic induced bleeding, the blood accumulates between the skull and the brain tissue. Aspiration of the hemorrhage is a relatively uncomplicated procedure and the prognosis for recovery is usually excellent. Return of brain function is complete.

In the event of spontaneous rupture, the collapse to the sidewalk would have occurred as consciousness was lost from bleeding within the brain. Often, neurosurgical removal of blood clots within the brain provides only temporary decompression of the brain. The likelihood for recovery is quite poor.

To those who were interested in knowing the circumstances of Atkins's death, knowledge of medication usage would be essential.

Particularly helpful would be information regarding either use or nonuse of a blood thinner (anticoagulant).

Atkins died nine days following admission and the surgical interventive procedure. An autopsy was not done.

Later Revelations

In February 2004 New York City's medical examiner let slip the information that Atkins's medical chart showed that he had suffered a heart attack, congestive heart failure, and high blood pressure before his death.[4] What's more, he weighed 258 pounds. That information was publicized by the *Wall Street Journal* after its news source, the Physician's Committee for Responsible Medicine, received, by transmission error, a copy of a postmortem report intended for Atkin's personal physician.

At 258 pounds the six-foot-tall Atkins would have been classified as obese. In response to that revelation, Atkins's widow, Veronica, and Stuart Trager, a physician consultant for the Atkins companies, contended that Atkins's weight ballooned in the hospital because of fluid retention. That explanation is surely far off the mark. The medical team at New York Weill-Cornell Center would not have allowed Atkins's fluid intake to be unbalanced. Further, the 258 pounds surely represented admission weight.

Now, Atkins could have developed heart failure and fluid retention during the days and weeks prior to the collapse on the sidewalk. But if so, why did he not institute pharmaceutical therapy? Until further information is released, Atkins, with a hospital weight of 258 pounds, must be considered to have been obese at the time of his death.

The information about heart attack, congestive heart failure, and high blood pressure came from review of the medical chart. An autopsy was not performed, the examiners report revealed, because of family objections to the procedure. The medical examiner conducted only an external exam and a review of Atkins's hospital records.

Veronica Atkins did issue a statement that added detail about her husband's health, acknowledging that he had "some progression of coronary artery disease" including "new blockage of a secondary artery."[5] The Physician's Committee for Responsible Medicine said that it decided to release the information because Atkins's "health history was used to promote his terribly unhealthy eating plan."

The Atkins Empire

In the months following Atkins's death, his companies continued business as usual, but the clock is winding down. For thirty years Atkins was a big influence on the behavior of Americans, overweight or otherwise. He stood the food pyramid on its head. He made fantastic claims that made his diet sound like an elixir. He was a great commercial success, but his unproven dietary approach deserves nothing but condemnation.

ADDITIONAL HIGH-FAT/LOW-FAT REPORTS

In May 2003 two additional studies that compared clinical effectivity of the high-fat low-carbohydrate (Atkins-type) and the low-fat high-carbohydrate diet appeared in the *New England Journal of Medicine*.[6] To the surprise of many nutritional pundits, volunteers who had been randomized to the Atkins-type diet showed slightly greater weight reduction than those in the low-fat group.

In one study, performed by the Department of Medicine at the Philadelphia Veterans Affairs Medical Center,[7] 132 obese subjects were enrolled for a six-month weight reduction and atherosclerosis risk factor trial. In the other, a joint effort of the researchers from four medical university centers,[8] the trial lasted twelve months. The latter study group numbered sixty-three. The average weight for the subjects in the six-month study was 288 pounds; for the twelve-month study, weight averaged 218 pounds.

For both studies the ability to draw conclusions about the relative efficacy and safety of either diet was limited by the large percentage of participants who were lost to follow-up. In the former study only 79 of the 132 subjects (60 percent) completed the six-month period of observation, while only 37 of the 63 subjects (59 percent) in the latter study participated to the end.

What can be concluded about those who dropped out? Did they dislike the diet? Were they disillusioned by their progress? Whatever might be the case, how should the dropouts be considered in the data analysis? The *NEJM* editorial referee was not able to provide an answer.[9]

If the statistical consideration was limited to those subjects who participated to the end: in the six-month trial, the high-fat low-carbohydrate dieters lost more weight and the difference was clinically significant. For the twelve-month trial, the high-fat low-carbohydrate dieters also showed a greater loss of weight at six-months, but at the twelve-month termination point, there was no longer a significant difference in the weight reduction of the two dietary groups.

For both studies the two diet groups received nutritional counseling, but some might argue that the medical support was not sufficiently intensive and supportive. For each dietary group in both studies, there was evidence of rebound over the course of the trial. The initial weight effect for the high-fat low-carbohydrate diet in the second study was no longer clinically significant at twelve months. The major disappointment, as the editorial referee pointed out,[10] was that the weight loss was small in relation to the amount of excess weight carried by subjects so obese. The second disappointment was that little, if any, change in the two most important atherogenic risk factors, cholesterol level and blood pressure, was achieved by any of the dietary groups that comprised the two studies.

The clinical effects of a diet regimen can be determined only if compliance is total and uncompromising. The fact that two-fifths of subjects in both trials dropped out of each study suggests that of those who remained enrolled to the end, compliance was low. The American Heart Association was not impressed by the findings of either study. Its longtime recommendation of a conventional, balanced diet rich in fruits and vegetables with 30 percent of calories from fat was not changed by the published reports in the *NEJM*. "Our recommendations are not changing" said Dr. Robert Bonow, its president.[11]

The American Heart Association might review its recommendations in regard to the necessity for total dietary commitment, nevertheless. In a January 2003 study published in the *Journal of the American College of Cardiology*,[12] the present-day, medication-oriented approach for managing an elevated cholesterol level within the blood (hypercholesteremia) was found to be wanting. What is required, the investigators found, is intensive lifestyle and dietary changes, too. A half century ago Kempner found that the dietary compliance must be uncompromising. Nothing has changed. Nowadays, 61 percent of US adults are overweight. As R. O. Bonow and R. H. Eckel expressed,[13] in a perspective regarding the *NEJM* reports:

> The recipe for effective weight loss is a combination of motivation, physical activity, and caloric restriction; maintenance of weight loss is a balance between caloric intake and physical activity, with lifelong adherence. For society as a whole, prevention of weight gain is the first step in curbing the increasing epidemic of overweight and obesity. Until further evidence is available regarding the long-term benefits of a low-carbohydrate approach, physicians should continue to recommend a healthy lifestyle that includes regular physical activity and a balanced diet.

Indeed. And one might add: nothing has changed since the DASH reports of 1997 and 2001. A diet that emphasizes fruits, vegetables, and low-fat dairy products; that include whole grains, poultry, fish, and nuts; that contains only small amounts of red meat, sweets, and sugar-containing beverages; that contains decreased amounts of total and saturated fat and cholesterol; and that contains no more than 1150 mg of sodium lowers blood pressure substantially both in people with hypertension and in those without hypertension, as compared to (1) the typical diet in the United States and, especially, (2) the Atkins and similar-type diets. The effect of a diet on one's blood pressure must always remain the primary consideration.

NOTES

1. Samaha, FF et al. A low-carbohydrate as compared with a low-fat diet in severe obesity. *New England Journal of Medicine* 2003;**348**: 2074–2081.

Foster, GD et al. A randomized trial of a low-carbohydrate diet for obesity. *New England Journal of Medicine* 2003;**348**:2082–2090.

2. Dr. Robert C. Atkins, author of controversial but best-selling diet books, is dead at 72. *New York Times*, April 18, 2003.

3. In July 2005, Lance Armstrong, eight years following his last chemotherapy session, won the Tour de France race for the seventh consecutive time, a feat that has been accomplished by no other.

4. http://www.snopes.com/medical/doctor/atkins.asp.

5. http://www.usatoday.com/life/people/2004-02-10-atkins_x.htm-73k.

6. Samaha, FF et al. A low-carbohydrate as compared with a low-fat diet in severe obesity. *New England Journal of Medicine* 2003; **348**:2074–2081.

Foster, GD et al. A randomized trial of a low-carbohydrate diet for obesity. *New England Journal of Medicine* 2003;**348**:2082–2090.

7. Ibid.

8. Ibid.

9. Ware, JH. Interpreting incomplete data in studies of diet and weight loss. *New England Journal of Medicine* 2003;**348**:2136–2137.

10. Ibid.

11. *Houston Chronicle*. May 22, 2003, p. 18A.

12. Sdringda, S et al. Combined intense lifestyle and pharmacologic lipid treatment further reduce coronary events and myocardial perfusion abnormalities compared with usual-care cholesterol-lowering drugs in coronary artery disease. *Journal of the American College of Cardiology* 2003;**41**:263–270.

13. Bonow, RO and Eckel, RH. Diet, obesity, and cardiovascular risk. *New England Journal of Medicine* 2003;**348**:2057–2058.

CHAPTER 12

LOW CARB, CONTINUED

The public's thirst for weight-reducing diets has been never ending. In late 2003 and throughout 2004, one of the *New York Times's* number one nonfictional best-sellers was *The South Beach Diet.*[1] Perusal of the text, authored by Arthur Agatston, MD, a cardiologist who practices in Miami Beach, Florida, gives one the impression that South Beach is only a step or two away from the American Heart Association–condemned Atkins diet, which simply means that one is closing his arteries and leaching his bones at a slightly slower rate. What amazes me is that desperate people continue to fall prey to low-carbohydrate food-restricted schemes such as Atkins's and Agatston's without questioning whether or not the diet is scientifically and nutritionally justifiable.

The secret to the South Beach Diet, according to the author, is that one will be eating only "good" carbohydrates and fats and will be avoiding the "bad" ones. The diet is supposed to cause permanent weight loss and to surpass cravings. One doesn't even have to exercise daily. Nor does daily sodium require restriction.

The South Beach Diet Web site states, "Our diet is distinguished by the absence of calorie counts; percentage of fats, carbs, and protein; or even portion control." The regimen consists, essentially, of three stages. Phase 1 (first two weeks) is an Atkins-type diet. Phase 2 adds back some carbohydrates. Phase 3—for the rest of your life—permits most things, except for a few restrictions.

The foods recommended by Agatston are the very ones condemned by heart associations and cancer societies worldwide as causing deadly and debilitating diseases. The recipes contain about 10 percent carbohydrate, 40 percent fat, and 50 percent protein (range: 30 to 70 percent). John McDougall, MD, a nutritional specialist, offers a stinging commentary to the South Beach Diet and should be referenced by those seeking more information.[2] In support of his remarks, McDougall offers extracts from the American Heart Association Nutrition Committee report in the October 9, 2001, issue of the journal *Circulation*:[3]

> High-protein diets typically offer wide latitude in protein food choices, are restrictive in other food choices (mainly carbohydrates), and provide structured eating plans. They also often promote misconceptions about carbohydrates, insulin resistance, ketosis, and fat-burning as mechanisms of action for weight loss. . . . High-protein diets are not recommended. . . . Individuals who follow these diets are at risk for . . . potential cardiac, renal, bone, and liver abnormalities overall.

Agatston's book debuted in April 2003 with a backdrop of unconventional marketing techniques that proved to be very successful. The plug that got sales in motion came two months later from comments in the *New Yorker* magazine.[4] Former president Bill Clinton was using the diet to help take off pounds.[5] Book sales jumped by twenty thousand a week following that announcement.

Sales continued on a fast track into 2004 despite cautionary remarks in the Tufts University *Health & Nutrition Letter*, in May 2004, and from nutritional experts interviewed that same month by Sanjay Gupta, MD, CNN medical correspondent. The Tufts nutritional letter offered precise criticism: "Disappointingly, *The South Beach Diet* is simply yet another version of a fad wrapped within a gimmick."[6] The newsletter went on to say that the diet was "based on fallacies replete with faulty science, glaring nutritional inaccuracies, contradictions, and claims of scientific evidence minus the actual evidence."

The Tufts letter skewered Agatston's offering with: "Like a lot of other weight-loss books, *The South Beach Diet* says the program 'has been scientifically studied' and 'proven effective,' then offers up not a single reference in a scientific journal. . . . *The South Beach Diet* gives some just-plain-weird advice, too: have ice cream instead of white bread because it's less fattening (if only!); a baked potato topped with low-fat cheese or sour cream is less fattening than a plain one; and don't drink beer because it leads directly to fat deposits on your belly (as if calories from particular food ended up at particular body parts and you could decide with your food choices where you're going to gain or lose weight)."

The CNN commentary with Dr. Gupta and the nutritional experts went like this:[7]

> *DR. SANJAY GUPTA*: Lot of concern about this [the South Beach Diet] . . . low-carb diet. Wahida [Wahida Karmally, director of nutrition at the Irving Center of Columbia University Medical Center], are the concerns overblown, do you think?
>
> *KARMALLY*: These are real concerns, because heart disease is the number one killer. And when you consume a diet that has lots of saturated fat and cholesterol, your LDL cholesterol, which is the bad cholesterol, will go up, and it increases your risk for heart

disease, and there are other dangers as well. Your blood pressure can go up because you're missing out on all these fruits, vegetables, and whole grains and low-fat dairies.

GUPTA: You're clearly not a fan. But Amy [Amy O'Connor, deputy editor of *Prevention* magazine], you know, Dr. Atkins, before he died, he actually studied at his center down in North Carolina, and said in fact cholesterol levels go down. You'd think they go up, but, in fact, they go down. What about that?

O'CONNOR: I think that's because when you lose weight, your cholesterol goes down.[8]

GUPTA: So what's wrong with that? You're losing weight.

O'CONNOR: Well, what's wrong with that, is that you're missing out on fruits and vegetables and all their phytonutrients [chemicals within fruits and vegetables] that actually protect us against disease. And there actually is a side effect to a lot of these low-carb foods that a lot of people don't talk about, which is gastrointestinal distress, which I've experienced firsthand taste-testing low-carb products.

GUPTA: Is that right? That just doesn't feel good. You know, it's interesting. Heidi Skolnik [nutritionist for the New York Giants and the School of American Ballet], both Dr. Agatston . . . and Dr. Atkins . . . cardiologists . . . and this is the diet they came up with. Why is it potentially harmful to heart disease patients?

SKOLNIK: [the lack of disease-fighting] phytonutritents.[9] We also have to look at immune markers, anti-inflammatory markers, beyond just cholesterol, in terms of what's going on. And without the phytonutrients, it's short-sighted.

GUPTA: One thing for sure, these diets are definitely here to stay. They've become really popular, a part of our diet culture.

Despite the criticism from nutritional specialists, sales of Agatston's book remained at a brisk pace. By June 2004 Agatston was sufficiently emboldened to strike a deal with Kraft Foods.

Kraft decided to promote some of its products with the South Beach Diet trademark—products that can be used, as Agatston said during the joint announcement, by people following the South Beach diet program.[10] "With 64% of adults in the US considered overweight and 46% on some form of diet last year, we are looking for innovative new ways to make weight management easier and more enjoyable," said Lance Friedman, Kraft senior vice president.

The press release went on to state: "Kraft Foods markets many of the world's food brands, including *Kraft* cheese, *Maxwell House* and *Jacobs* coffees, *Philadelphia* cream cheese, *Oscar Mayer* meats, *Boca* products, *Balance* bars, and *Post* cereals in more than 150 countries."

Three of the Phase 1 South Beach Diet–Kraft meal plans were offered. The day 2 entry is shown below.

Breakfast:

Crustless Country Quiche (cholesterol-free egg product, *Boca* Meatless Breakfast Links, asparagus spears, *Knudsen* Low-Fat Cottage Cheese, *Kraft* Reduced-Fat Cheddar Cheese, onion, *Grey Poupon* Dijon Mustard)

2 *Boca* Breakfast Links

6 oz vegetable juice

6 oz *Maxwell House* Decaffeinated Coffee

Snack:

1 oz *Planters* Almonds—Plain

8 oz *Crystal Light* (Peach Iced Tea)

Lunch:

Cobb Lettuce Wraps (lettuce, *Louis Rich* Turkey Bacon, *Oscar Mayer* Smoked Turkey Breast, avocado, tomato, *Kraft Carbwell Roka* Blue Cheese Dressing)

5 cherry tomatoes

½ cup raw red pepper slices

½ cup celery sticks

1 cup broth

8 oz skim milk

Snack:

Sun-Dried Tomato and Cheese Dip (*Polly-O* Natural Part-Skim Ricotta Cheese, *Kraft* 100% Grated Parmesan Cheese, sun-dried tomatoes, vinegar, salt, green onions)

½ cup raw broccoli

½ cup raw cauliflower

Dinner:

Salmon with Tomatoes, Spinach and Mushrooms (with *Kraft Carbwell* Light Italian Dressing)

Feta and Vegetable Grill (zucchini, tomato, green pepper, onion, *Athenos* Crumbled Reduced-Fat Feta Cheese, olive oil)

½ cup sliced avocado

Tossed salad (mixed greens, cucumbers, cherry tomatoes, green peppers)

¼ cup kidney beans

2 tbsp *Carbwell* Salad Dressing—Light Buttermilk Ranch

8 oz skim milk

Dessert:

Creamy Gelatin Layered Squares (*Jell-O* Brand Lime Flavor Low-Calorie Gelatin, water, *Cool Whip Lite* Whipped Topping)

Polly-O Reduced Fat Mozzarella cheese stick

Nutrient content (Kraft saved one the trouble of doing the arithmetic):

Calories	1630
Total Fat (g)	78
Saturated Fat (g)	20
Cholesterol (mg)	350
Carbohydrate (g)	101
Protein (g)	124
Sodium (mg)	3780

Quick calculation shows that a whooping 44 percent of calories come from fat. And notice the staggering 3780 mg of sodium.

Certain Kraft foods, Agatston noted in Web site commentary, meet the nutritional principles of the South Beach Diet.[11] Those products will be labeled with a circular blue button that reads "South Beach Diet™ Recommended." They include lean Oscar Mayer meats, Kraft reduced-fat cheese, and Boca meat substitutes. Never mind that those products still contain an abundance of fat and that sodium content will be quite high. Agatston and Kraft Foods had found each other.

In January 2004 Clinton acknowledged that he was adhering to the South Beach Diet and that he had lost fifteen pounds.[12] Earlier, he went on to say, he had tried the Atkins diet but was unable to maintain the weight loss.

A few months later, though, Clinton began experiencing ominous symptoms—shortness of breath and angina (chest pain). Upon leaving the White House in 2001, his blood pressure was mildly elevated and his "bad" LDL cholesterol was 134 in comparison to the desired upper limit of 100.[13]

The onset of angina indicated that immediate cardiovascular workup was necessary. That evaluation took place at Westchester Medical Center near Clinton's home. Among the battery of initial tests that were performed, the LDL cholesterol was found to be elevated to 177, an alarming jump of 43 points. A cholesterol-lowering medication was begun immediately, and a blood pressure medication was required as well.[14]

The supposition that adherence to the South Beach Diet can maintain blood cholesterol at a safe level, a proposition espoused by Agatston, was immediately laid to rest. The loss of fifteen pounds was laudable, but control of the blood pressure and the LDL cholesterol deserved greater concern.

Apparently, Clinton did not realize that excess weight and elevated LDL cholesterol require independent management. A reduction in calories consumed along with an increase in calories burned during exercise produces weight loss. Blood cholesterol reduction requires low-fat dietary regimentation as Kempner[15] demonstrated many years ago. That's the nutritional principle that Atkins refused to believe and that Agatston does not seem to appreciate.

Consider that a ten-year study of 4,047 severely obese individuals in Sweden showed no decrease in blood cholesterol level following bariatric (stomach reduction) surgery.[16] Weight loss, on the other hand, was considerable. At the two-year interval, the loss amounted to 23.4 percent of initial body weight. At ten years, the loss was somewhat less, at 16.1 percent. During that period of time the diet mix of carbohydrate, fat, and protein preferred by each trial subject was not altered and as a result the concentration of cholesterol in the bloodstream remained unchanged.

Next, in the Clinton cardiovascular workup, was coronary arteriography, a minor operative procedure during which a catheter is inserted into an artery within the groin so that a radiopaque dye can be injected within the coronary arteries and the flow studied by x-ray. The procedure is performed in hospitals, nowadays, 600,000 times a year.[17] For Clinton, arteriography revealed severe coronary artery blockage from cholesterol deposition—as much as 90 percent closure for some of the arteries.[18] The involvement was too severe for balloon dilatation and stent insertion. Instead, Clinton was transferred to New York Presbyterian Hospital/Columbia where, after a short delay, successful quadruple bypass surgery was performed.

Following news of Clinton's troubles, weekly sales of *The South Beach Diet* slowed to about twenty thousand copies in early October, down from seventy thousand a few weeks earler.[19] "The bloom is off the rose," said Bob Goldin, executive vice president of the food industry consulting firm Technomic. "It doesn't look like the market has any staying power."[20]

A short time following his discharge from the hospital, Clinton acknowledged, on ABC's *Primetime Live* program, that he wished he had forgone the recent low-carb regimen of steaks and cheeseburgers in favor of a diet devoid of fat.[21] At the same time it was divulged that his wife, Hillary, had been worried that his low-carb high-protein diet was unhealthy before onset of cardiac decompensation in September 2004, but he had shrugged off her fears.[22]

By late 2004 it was obvious that the general public had learned from the difficulties that Clinton had encountered. Disenchantment with low-carb food products had taken a toll on high-profile Atkins Nutritionals, Inc., the marketing firm that Robert Atkins, MD, founded in 1989. As the *New York Times* reported, Atkins Nutritionals, Inc. was forced to write off $53 million in unsold and expired food in late 2004. The company's quarterly revenues had dropped from $87 million in January 2004 to $29 million in August.[23] In October 2004, Atkins Nutritionals, Inc. acknowledged that it had hired a turnaround specialist and that it was cutting jobs.[24] Don't pity Atkins's surviving spouse, Veronica. She sold controlling interest in Atkins Nutritionals, Inc. to Pantheon Capital and Goldman Sachs in October 2003 for a reported $533 million.[25]

In July 2005 Atkins Nutritionals, Inc. commenced bankruptcy proceedings.

NOTES

1. http://www.medicinet.com/script/main/art.asp?articlekey=40936-31K-.

2. http://www.drmcdougall.com/new/south_beach_diet.html.

3. St. Jear, S. Dietary protein and weight reduction: a statement for healthcare professionals from the Nutrition Committee of the Council on Nutrition, Physical Activity, and Metabolism of the American Heart Association. *Circulation* 2001;**104**:1869–1974.

4. http://www.fitfaq.com/2004/06/south-beach-diets-journey-to-the-top.html.

5. Clinton and five hundred other celebrities had been sent a copy of *The South Beach Diet* by Rodale, the publisher.

6. Weighing in on *the South Beach Diet*. Tufts *Health and Nutrition Letter*. May 2004.

7. http://transcripts.cnn.com/TRANSCRIPTS/0405/21/ltm.01.html.

8. Not necessarily. Cholesterol will decrease only if dietary fat as

well as dietary calories are reduced. See comments, page 229, regarding weight reduction with bariatric surgery.

9. Example: phytonutrients would be lycopene, in tomatoes particularly, and flavenoids, in berries.

10. Kraft Foods and Dr. Arthur Agatston form alliance to help people eat and live better. Kraft will use South Beach Diet trademark to promote certain products. Northfield, IL, June 9, 2004. See http://kraft.com/newsroom/060904.html.

11. http://www.southbeachdiet.com.

12. http://www/hollandsentinel.com/stories/011604.

13. http://www.edition.cnn.com/TRANSCRIPTS/0406/06/ltm.04 html-52k-.

14. http://www.supermarketguru.com/page.cfm/9096.

15. Kempner, W. Radical dietary treatment of hypertensive and arteriosclerotic vascular disease, heart and kidney disease, and vascular retinopathy. *GP* 1954;**IX**:71–93.

16. Sjöström L, Lindroos AK, et al. Lifestyle, diabetes and cardiovascular risk factors 10 years after bariatric surgery. *New England Journal of Medicine* 2004;**351**:2683–2693.

17. Most common diagnoses and procedures in US community hospitals. http://www.ahrg.gov/date/hcup/commdx/table2a.htm-43k-.

18. http://www.dadtalk.typepad.com/dadtalk/health/index.html.

19. Nielson Book Scan. Quoted by MSNBC News. December 11, 2004.

20. MSNBC News. December 11, 2004.

21. ABC News Original Report. October 28, 2004. How Clinton recovered from surgery.

22. http://momosearch.com/directory/heart-healthy-diet-plan.html.

23. Warner, Melanie. Is the low-carb boom over? Sunday Business *New York Times*. December 5, 2004, p. 1.

24. Corel, S and Toll, D. Atkins Nutritionals trimming work force. Dow Jones Newswires. http://www.thestate.com/mld/thestate/business/9634797.html-27k-.

25. http://www.medicalnewstoday.com/index.php?newsid=7400-32k-.

CHAPTER 13

WALTER KEMPNER AND NATHAN PRITIKIN

It would be difficult to conclude a text of this type without special recognition of Walter Kempner and Nathan Pritikin who, each in his own way, put the rationale for dietary therapy on a sound basis and devised the course of implementation.

WALTER KEMPNER, MD

Walter Kempner is one of those individuals whose stature is likely to grow over time. When he died in 1997, at age ninety-three, recognition of his lifetime accomplishments appeared in the local press only. Those who had known Kempner and who were aware of his extraordinary achievements in the management of kidney, heart, and blood vessel diseases of all types were surprised, surely, that the recognition had not been disseminated further. After all, Kempner had been the pioneer, fifty years before, of low-fat, low-

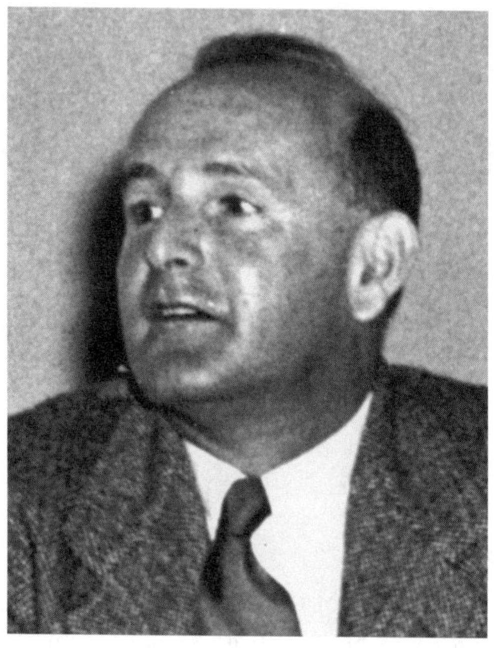

Walter Kempner (1903–1997), circa 1954.

protein, and low-sodium dietary therapy for circulatory problems of all sorts. Beginning in the 1940s and continuing almost until his death, Kempner had presided, at Duke University School of Medicine in Durham, North Carolina, over the care of thousands of desperately ill patients.

In 1934 Duke recruited Kempner from Berlin's Kaiser Wilhelm Institute of Cellular Physiology. His field of research was oxidative and fermentative metabolism, which he conducted in the laboratory of Otto Warburg, the 1931 Nobel laureate in cellular physiology. Subsequent to Kempner's relocation in North Carolina, as a Jewish émigré from Nazi Germany, his cellular physiological studies resumed and, in time, extended to a variety of tissues, most notable of which was the kidney.[1] That latter work led to the consideration of what could be done for renal metabolic dysfunction (kidney disease) and, in 1939–40, to his introduction of a revolutionary therapeutic dietary regimen, in time to become known as the rice/fruit diet.

Initially, Kempner introduced his low-fat, low-protein, and low-sodium diet solely for management of kidney disease. Calories totaled from 1,000 to 2,400. For 2,000 calories, less than 40 came from fat and only 80 from protein. Sodium was restricted to 250 mg.

The rice/fruit and sodium-restricted regimen was prescribed to desperately ill patients for a period of days or weeks. By 1942 Kempner found that remarkable results could be obtained by continuing the diet long term. Kidney function could be ameliorated, and equally impressive was the remarkable improvement in the circulatory status of his patients. Next, he began managing patient after patient, in the 1940s, with high blood pressure, which was often of very severe degree. The results were impressive, if not astounding. No one had ever before salvaged patients with malignant high blood pressure. In time, Kempner extended his dietary therapy to patients with heart failure, advanced-stage diabetes mellitus, and, finally, to those with obesity.

At the 1944 annual meeting of the American Medical Association, results were presented that documented decrease in heart size, improved kidney function, and reversal of retinopathy following institution of the Kempner dietary regimen.[2] The consensus among medical professionals had been that dietary therapy was of no value in kidney, blood vessel, and heart diseases. A leading textbook of the time stated, "No dietary treatment is known which has a specifically favorable effect on essential hypertension."[3] Another said: "The diet in uncomplicated hypertension requires no essential change from the normal. There is no justification for restriction of protein intake; indeed, such restriction may result in anemia, and other evidences of malnutrition. Likewise, in the absence of edema or paroxysmal dyspnea, the restriction of salt is unwarranted."[4]

Although skepticism prevailed, patients with heart and blood vessel diseases learned of the new treatment that offered hope and flocked to Kempner's Duke University clinic. Rather quickly the medical center was transformed from a university hospital that offered local services to an internationally known institution for the treatment of circulatory diseases.

Kempner found that in order to achieve the results he desired, dietary compliance must be total. The advice he extended to his patients was uncompromising. Compliance that is simply, in his words, "fat-poor, salt-poor and protein-poor," would have only limited therapeutic possibilities. "One should wage total war," he often said.

Kempner's greatest triumphs came in the management of malignant hypertension, a dramatic, short-term disease with a high mortality rate. He was able to demonstrate reversibility. For those with elevated serum cholesterol, he showed that diet would lower the level significantly. He found that xanthoma, a tumorous-like fat deposit beneath the skin surface, could be reversed with diet therapy. If coronary artery perfusion studies had been performed at that time, Kempner surely would have demonstrated cholesterol plaque dissolution, too. That revelation was left to Ornish and his coworkers to document many years later,[5] in patients with such a problem who adhered to the rigorous dietary regimen for two years or more.

Kempner showed that his patients became insulin-sensitive and that the dose of insulin required by diabetic patients was decreased by a low-fat, low-protein, and low-sodium dietary regimen. Many endocrinologists found that revelation hard to accept for the prevailing, and mistaken, wisdom had been, and still is to some degree even today, that carbohydrates must be restricted in the diabetic diet. In 1945 Kempner published his first retinal photographs showing the disappearance of exudates and hemorrhages in the diabetic patient.[6] In 1958 a paper "Effect of Rice Diet on Diabetes Mellitus Associated with Vascular Disease" reported on one hundred patients with diabetes mellitus treated by the rice diet.[7] Reversibility of diabetic retinopathy was demonstrated (figs. 1 and 2). But most ophthalmologists remained oblivious of his accomplishments because the reports were placed only in journals for general medical physicians.

Kempner treated patients with kidney diseases of all types. His results, outstanding by any measure, were thought to be exaggerated and, as a result, were simply dismissed by many medical profes-

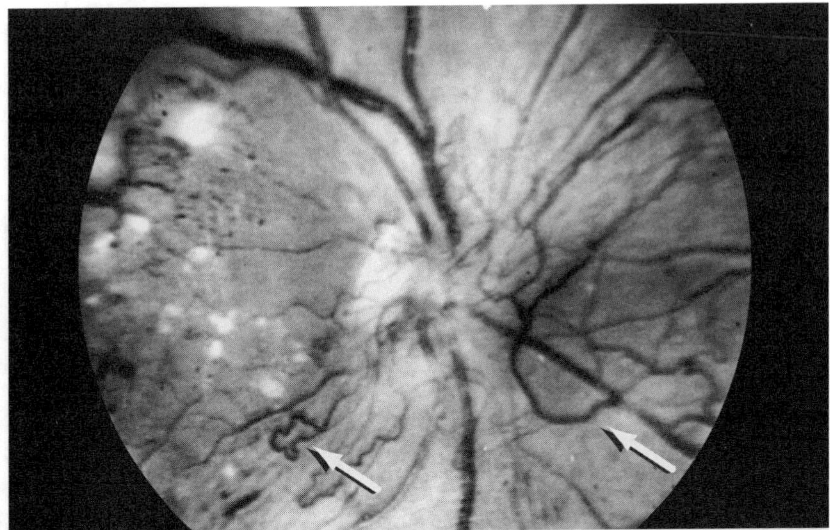

Fig. 1. Complete reversal of nervehead neovascularization in diabetes mellitus—an extraordinary development!—following thirty-five-month adherence to rice/fruit and 250 mg sodium-restricted diet. Note bizarre, newly proliferating blood vessels near the nervehead (arrows) and their subsequent regression. Right eye of BC, female, age thirty-eight. (Photographs courtesy of Barbara Newborg, MD, custodian of Kempner's records)

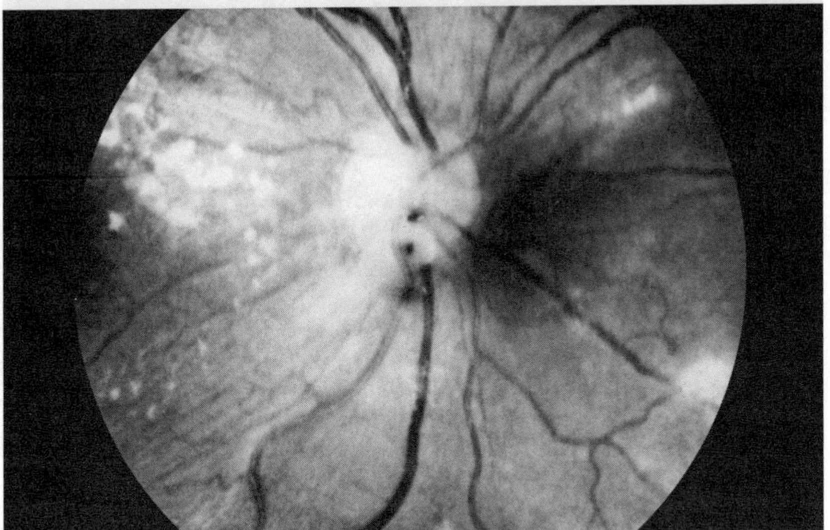

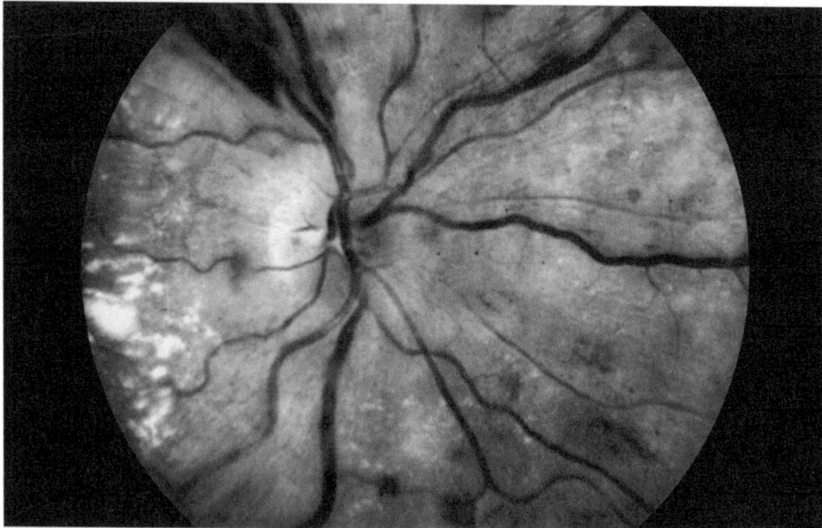

Fig. 2. Kempner's patient, FF, a twenty-eight-year-old female with an eighteen-year history of diabetes mellitus. August 1950 photograph of right eye showed advanced neovascular stage diabetic retinopathy. Rice/fruit–250 mg Na diet was begun. June 1953: Marked regression of diabetic retinopathy is apparent. (Photos courtesy of Barbara Newborg, MD, custodian of Kempner's records)

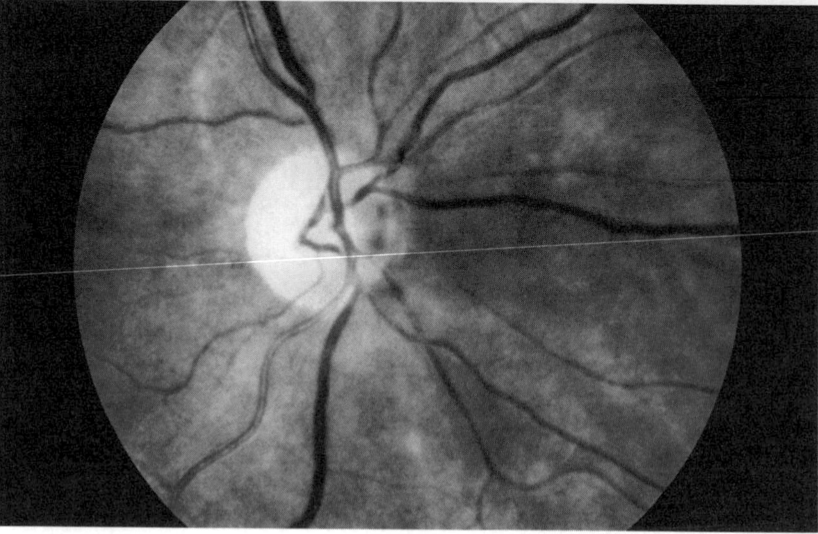

sionals. He was soundly criticized because he had not performed control trials. Those who were able to observe firsthand were impressed, nevertheless. "For those with kidney disease," said Eugene Stead in 1974,[8] the illustrious and much-respected chief of internal medicine at Duke, "the edema, hypercholesteremia, hyperproteinemia, and hypertension responded well [to the Kempner regimen]." Then, in further defense of Kempner, Stead noted, "He demonstrated that nephrotic children wasting large amounts of protein [also] did well on the rice diet. The proteinuria decreased dramatically and the children showed good growth." "It is of interest to consider why Kempner has received in this country little recognition for his tremendous achievement," Dr. Stead went on to say. "He did not appeal to the scientific community. It wanted him to set up various kinds of control studies. He contended that each patient was his own control and that there were already enough studies of patients treated by other forms of therapy. He was unwilling to deny any of his patients the full benefit of what he thought was best."

Kempner used his diet for all patients with hypertension, heart failure, renal failure, diabetes, and obesity. He recognized that to be overweight was as serious a disease as diabetic retinopathy. Stead finished his appraisal of Kempner with: "Things are more black and white in Kempner's mind than in the mind of most physicians."

Kempner was totally devoted to his patients. He wanted/demanded good results. Stead again:

> He treated all forms of vascular disease—mild, intermediate, and severe. He was not concerned about the patient's symptoms. The patient's physician at home knew that the vascular disease was in many instances not the cause of the complaining. When the patient returned home after three months of rigid therapy directed at an asymptomatic disease, the physician saw red. But in Kempner's defense, for many years he saw more destructive vas-

> cular disease than any other physician. In many instances, the disease destroyed the patient in spite of everybody's best efforts. It is little wonder that Kempner treated mild disease seriously.

Stead attempted to justify Kempner's actions this way:

> He has made many enemies because he has been honest and uncompromising and has never spent a single hour of his life, except for some scientific talks on rare occasions, in any society or even in a committee meeting.

In the 1950s, diuretics, medications that stimulate kidney excretion of sodium, were introduced for the management of high blood pressure. Never mind that diuretics also caused the kidney to excrete potassium, a most essential electrolyte, pill therapy for hypertension was readily accepted by both the medical profession and the patients all too willingly to avoid the rigors of a low-sodium diet. The potassium deficit could be countered by taking, it was felt, a supplement (another tablet).

During the last decades of Kempner's life as newer drug therapies became available, the direct application of his dietary regimen diminished as a large array of blood pressure medications—Beta blockers, ACE inhibitors, angiotensin antagonists, and calcium channel blockers—became available for the management of hypertension. Reference to an alternative such as the Kempner regimen was avoided.

Most recently, some medical physicians have begun to suspect that the pendulum has swung too far in the direction of drug therapy. Ornish has suggested that the initial approach for relief of a medical problem be directed at causation.[9] Assuming that the present-day flip-flop in dietary electrolytes is responsible for most high blood pressure cases—now numbering fifty million in the United States—

should not the initial therapeutic step be dietary rehabilitation? For Kempner, medications were always a choice of last resort.

Emeritus Status

In 1972 at age sixty-nine Kempner became an emeritus professor at Duke. Honors finally began to come his way. The *Archives of Internal Medicine* published a Kempner symposium. In 1975 he was given the Ciba[10] award for hypertension research. In 1979 a Walter Kempner professorship was established at Duke University. In 1983 the German Bundespraesident conferred the Grosse Verdienstkrenz (highest Order of Merit) on Kempner.

After Kempner became professor emeritus he continued his practice at an off-campus facility, the Rice House, until his retirement in 1992. In 1997 he died in his sleep after having experienced no premonitory symptoms. He had never married. Eight million dollars of his estate was designated to establish annuities for a few of his associates with the provision that upon the death of each, the principal would become available to Duke University Medical School.[11]

Stefan George Disciple

Kempner's body was cremated and the ashes were sent by mail to Minusio, Switzerland, and, in accordance with his will, buried near Stefan George,[12] Germany's most respected intellectual during the first third of the twentieth century. The latter lived from 1868 to 1933. In his early years, George was Germany's most influential poet and today easily ranks with Goethe, Hölderin, or Rilke. In the early 1900s George gathered round himself a group of scholars who espoused an elitist and hierarchical ideology. The circle of disciples expressed contempt for Germany's democratic experiment that followed the First

World War and instead provided a surrogate philosophy that looked back to a heroic European past for cultural and political models.

Many esteemed writers, including Friedrich Gundolf and Karl Wolfskehl, belonged to the George circle, as the group was called. George's influence grew steadily and by 1929, according to one newspaper account, he was "one of six contemporary figures who have [already] become legends." The others, whose likenesses were featured along with George's in the newspaper account, were Woodrow Wilson, Georges Clemenceau, Hindenburg, Gandhi, and Lenin. George was the only one who was not a professional politician.

While working at the Kaiser Wilhelm Institute and the Berlin Charite Hospital, Kempner found time to assume the role of personal physician to Stefan George. The latter had a frail constitution during the last few years of his life. His physical status had been compromised by bladder surgery for stone removal in 1925 and, one can reasonably conclude, by his lifelong cigarette-smoking habit.

That Kempner could find time to assume a physician-patient responsibility to George is witness to the former's energetic disposition. From 1927 to 1935, following graduation from the University of Heidelberg Medical School in 1926, Kempner authored (or provided supervision for) nine papers that appeared in scientific publications. He had been introduced into the Stefan circle in 1922, at age nineteen.

On January 30, 1933, President Hindenburg handed over the reins of the German government to Adolf Hitler, who would come close to destroying it. That action followed intense negotiations between the two during which Hitler was able to convince Hindenburg that the Nazi Party under Hitler's leadership as chancellor of Germany would restore the country to good health.

In May 1933 the new minister for science, art, and education, as spokesman for Joseph Goebbels, the propaganda minister, attempted to establish a favorable allegiance with George by way of a Writers'

Academy that was being formed. As it was explained to George, "The ministry wants to describe you to the press as forefather of the current government." At the same time, Nazi Germany was beginning its upheaval. On April 1 a national boycott of Jewish shops and businesses was put into effect. On April 7 the government enacted a decree known as the Reestablishment Law of the Civil Service, which had the effect of excluding Jews from civil service, university, and state positions. And on May 10 public demonstrations that included the burning of books written by Jews, political dissidents, and others not approved by the state were held in several cities.

George was nauseated by such actions and all that was implied by them. Several of the more esteemed members of his circle were Jewish. His reply to the Goebbels proposal read as follows: "In short: I can accept no post—even an honorary one." And, "for almost half a century I have administered German literature and German spirit without an academy—indeed had there been one probably [I would have been] against it."[13]

To escape the inclement Berlin winters, George spent much of the winters of 1931–32 and 1932–33 in Minusio. Then, as the actions of the new government—the Third Reich—unfolded in the summer of 1933, George again left Germany and went to Switzerland. In 1952 his personal attorney and longtime circle member, Ernst Morwitz, who was Jewish, explained, George's actions this way: "[His was] an unambiguous protest against totalitarian compulsion and the increasing misinterpretation of his ideas and words. He left the country and spent the rest of his life in exile."[14] He had been reluctant to return to Berlin in the spring of 1932 and, again, in spring 1933; what he would have done in 1934 cannot be known for sure.

In contemporary life George had looked toward the rise of supermen who would unify the state and culture. By the summer of 1933 the divergence of those aesthetic ideals and the brutalized reality of the Third Reich had become all too apparent.

The stay in Switzerland in 1933 would last only three months. In September George's physical condition took a turn for the worse. He became noticeably weak and tired. By mid-October his status had become grave. He died on December 4. Kempner was at his bedside. One who aided the supportive effort and directed the death vigil was twenty-six-year-old Claus von Stauffenberg, a member of the George circle since 1923. Following George's death, Stauffenberg, as well as some other non-Jewish members of the circle, signed on (in 1935, in Stauffenberg's case) with the Nazi cause. Stauffenberg fought in the Second World War from the first campaigns onward, taking part in the invasion of Poland in September 1939 and in the western offensive in France the following year. As a tank commander he earned the reputation of being a highly effective leader who was valued for organizational skills, discipline, and courage.

By late 1941 Stauffenberg's appraisal of the hostilities had changed. He became appalled by the indifference of the German high command toward human life, as innumerable Jewish peasants in Russia were rounded up and shot and as an equal number of Russian soldiers died miserable deaths in captivity. About the same time he received information that a camp called Auschwitz had been established to burn Jews in ovens. To a close friend he said, "They are shooting Jews on a massive scale. These crimes should not be permitted to continue."[15]

Stauffenberg and some other like-minded officers formed a group of conspirators to remove Hitler from power. That action culminated in an attempt to kill the Führer on July 20, 1944. During a staff meeting at Hitler's headquarters, Stauffenberg, whose rank in 1944 was that of colonel, placed a briefcase of explosives under a wooden map table around which a strategy session was being conducted. The bomb exploded but Hitler, though injured, survived. Stauffenberg was arrested and executed by firing squad. In personal documents that had been composed prior to the assassination attempt, and which were discovered after the war, it was apparent that Stauffenberg had remained loyal to the ideals he had learned from Stefan George.

Others of the George circle, including Kempner, left Germany before the World War II cataclysm. Kempner's brother, Robert, a civil servant attorney and not a member of the George circle, escaped in 1935. He came to the United States and later enlisted in the army, where he served in the intelligence corps. Following the conclusion of hostilities, he served as deputy prosecutor in the 1946 Nuremberg trials of war criminals.

Albert Einstein, the Kaiser Wilhelm Institute's most revered professor (of physics), left Berlin in December 1932 and made his way to the newly created Institute for Advanced Study in Princeton, New Jersey. Kempner left his beloved Germany and the Kaiser Wilhelm Institute in 1934. But far too few would be able to take advantage of the brief interval for exodus.

Unique Medical Practitioner

Kempner had been destined for medical fame from the time he was born. His parents were respected scientists in their time, and both were members of the Koch Institute. His father discovered a cure for botulism and his mother made important contributions in the bacteriological study of tuberculosis. She was the first woman professor in Germany as a result of having established the pathogenicity of bovine tuberculosis for humans. Her discovery led to the decision to slaughter tuberculosis-infected cows with the ultimate effect of saving hundreds of Berlin children.

The picture that emerges of Kempner's medical practice at Duke University is that he was a brilliant physician who demanded discipline and loyalty from associates and patients. He was known for an authoritarian bedside manner that surely had been styled after Stefan George's demeanor. Further, Kempner (like George) surrounded himself with faithful and devoted associates, some of whom he brought from Germany.

He patterned his lifestyle after George's—the leader image, the devoted associates, the unwavering sense of discipline. His hospital manner deviated from the norm. He did not hesitate to scold patients when they were not complying with his instructions. He would even threaten to remove them from the program if they deviated repeatedly from the dietary regimen. He thought the risk to their lives was so great that his demeanor warranted harshness.

His medical practice was tarnished by one unfortunate incident. In 1975 allegations regarding Kempner's use of a whip came out in a lawsuit filed by a former employee. When Duke University officials heard about the whippings, they were shocked. He was told to leave the medical center.

The exile was not a hardship since Kempner could, and did, continue his practice elsewhere in Durham. His staff and patients still used the Duke facilities. Kempner seemed surprised that his behavior caused an uproar. Later, he said, "I have whipped people (on the rare occasion, as it was) to help them and because they said they want to be whipped."[16]

If Kempner was bitter toward Duke University because of his treatment, he didn't show it. Several months before his death he designated most of his estate in planned annuity arrangements for his associates and Duke. Included in his bequeath to the university were rare manuscripts and books that had once belonged to Friedrich Gundolf (1880–1931), a classics scholar and one of George's most gifted and devoted followers.

Cellular Physiologist

After Kempner became settled at Duke, the outpouring of cellular physiology papers continued. Between 1936 and 1939, the number of peer-reviewed publications was twenty. Otto Warburg, his mentor in Berlin, had developed apparati and methods by which reactions of living cells could be studied under various conditions and with various substrates. Kempner conducted studies with normal cells in a physiological milieu. He found that oxygen tension played a significant role in cellular metabolism.

His studies with laboratory-propagated kidney cells led to the conclusion that a diet with the virtual elimination of sodium and fat and only a minimal amount of protein would provide the most desirable milieu for a person with a diseased kidney. His regimen would provide, additionally, high potassium levels and low chloride. The diet lived up to its promise, and it also provided unanticipated results: decrease in heart size, compensation of heart and kidney failure, restoration of eyesight, and reversal of diabetes mellitus.[17]

NATHAN PRITIKIN

"All I'm trying to do is wipe out heart disease, diabetes, hypertension, and obesity." That statement personified Nathan Pritikin's mission. And the zeal with which he undertook that mission touched off a war between Pritikin and the medical establishment that abated only during the last year or two of his life.

Pritikin[18] was born on Chicago's West Side on August 29, 1915. His parents were eastern European Jews who had come to the United States as infants with their parents. His father's family arrived from Kiev, Ukraine (Russia), in 1891. His mother's family came from Poland. Both families settled in predominately Jewish neighborhoods.

In 1933 Nathan entered the University of Chicago on a scholarship. At the same time he managed a photography business with his brother. They specialized in photographing banquets, conventions,

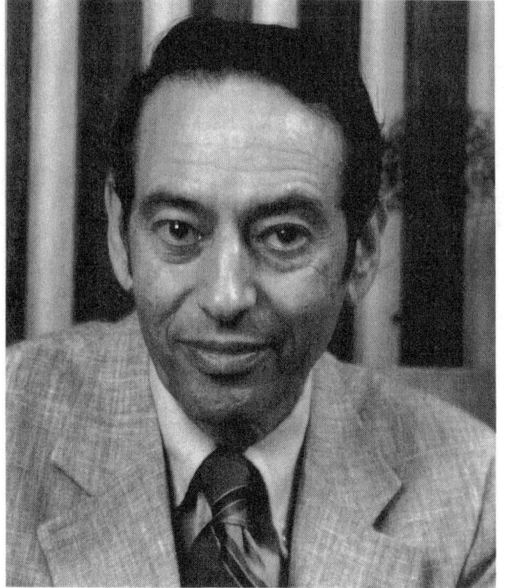

Nathan Pritikin (1915–1985), circa 1972.

baseball teams, and social clubs. The business was an outstanding success despite the fact that the US economy was mired in a depression. In 1935 young Pritikin discontinued his studies to devote more time to the photography business.

He was inventive. He was able to devise cameras of special type for various purposes. When World War II commenced, his interests turned to instrumentation that could enable the war effort. One challenge was the Nordham bombsight. He was able to improve the reticules used by the bombardier. A large contract was obtained with the air force and his fifty-person staff became overwhelmed with orders.

Interest in Medicine

In his early teens Pritikin took an interest in medicine. He learned the names of all 206 bones in the human body. Many days were spent studying exhibits at Chicago's Field Museum of Natural History. Medical conferences were also of special interest to Pritikin. In those early days, his photography assignments were often medical groups. Whenever he was presented with the opportunity, he took an empty seat in the banquet room and listened intently as doctors lectured on everything from brain surgery to heart disease and proctology.

Relocation in California

In 1955 Pritikin moved his family, several tons of equipment, and ten key employees to Santa Barbara, California. He felt that business opportunities would be plentiful on the West Coast and that the mild climate would benefit both his family and his business.

Over the next several years, he developed several businesses in addition to Phototronics, his flagship company. One company made high-precision dies and die-stamped metal parts. Another made optical encoders, by which commands were transmitted to automated machines and computers. Still another produced retractable, porous-tipped pens. A final company produced measuring instruments.

Phototronics, which evolved from his initial business enterprise in Chicago, produced electronic devices and printed circuits, including the circuit boards in handheld calculators and in memory banks for computers. Phototronics employed 150 people.

He was brilliant. More than nineteen US and twenty-four foreign patents were issued in his name in fields as diverse as engineering and aeronautics. His inventions included a new method for making inlaid circuits that were flush with their insulation base (patented in 1954); a new method for making printed circuits (patented in 1955); an improved electrical resistor and the technology for producing them inexpensively (1958), which was followed by several other improved versions, all of which were patented through the 1960s; thin films that were used as electrical conductors and the technology to produce them (1964); a new process for embedding circuits in insulated bases, making them resistant to heat and moisture, and protecting them from shock; and better inlaid circuits and methods for producing them (1965).

Soon after he became settled in California, he sought out an internal medicine physician for a thorough health examination. His cholesterol count was 280 mg/dl and his EKG showed early evidence of heart disease. And while his physician was not too alarmed, Pritikin was much too knowledgeable of medical diseases to know that the findings should not be casually dismissed.

Even as he worked twelve- to fifteen-hour days developing his businesses, Pritikin had maintained a keen interest in medicine. So, when he learned about his elevated cholesterol, he had an inkling about what must be done to restore his body to good health. That approach would necessitate a radical change in dietary habits. In 1958, and continuing for the next ten years, Pritikin kept meticulous track of his health as he made daring changes in his diet. For weeks on end his diet was vegetarian—whole grains, vegetables, and fruits. Next, he would change the proportions of these foods and simply add beef or fish or poultry for a week. His cholesterol level fell with the dietary changes. From the 280 mg/dl high the cholesterol dropped steadily to 102 mg/dl by December 1963. When rice was eliminated and substituted with a serving of meat per day, the cholesterol level crept up to 158 mg/dl. From there his cholesterol declined to 118 mg/dl after he discontinued meat.

Particularly gratifying was the improvement in the EKG tracing. By 1959 the recording had regained a normal configuration for all leads.

Interests Turn to Health

Pritikin's medical interests had been aroused and he soon gained an encyclopedic knowledge of general health, nutritional, and medical subjects. His recovery left him with a feeling of rebirth. He exercised daily. Conventional wisdom at the time was that a person with heart disease should be temperate in all things. Excessive exercise was to be avoided. Dietary constraints were thought to have little or no effect on heart disease. The caloric composition of the average US diet at the time contained 40 to 45 percent fat.

Emboldened by the results of his dietary and exercise program, Pritikin's passionate study of health, nutrition, and medicine began to completely overtake him. He subscribed to several medical journals. His personal library of medical textbooks grew and grew. Gradually, he turned the daily operation of his companies over to management and devoted his attention to the study of health.

People began to seek him out for medical advice. Most of these clients suffered from forms of heart disease, such as coronary insufficiency, angina, or high blood pressure. Others had adult-onset diabetes, and still others suffered from gout, kidney stone and gallstones, arthritis, and claudication (deficient circulation in the legs). He provided all advice for free.

By 1971 his understanding of medical problems had reached a point that he collaborated with two local Santa Barbara scientists in writing *Live Longer Now*,[19] a treatise documenting the relationship of diet to the leading diseases. By this time the body of information that he had accumulated filled two rooms of his house.

The text addressed each illness in a standardized structure. Biological mechanisms causing the disease were explained and then the role of diet for reversal of the disease. The introduction to the text began with four inciteful paragraphs:

> The various degenerative diseases—atherosclerosis, including coronary heart disease, hypertension, diabetes, cancer, glaucoma and arthritis—proceed relentlessly to claim many millions of victims. If not fatal, these diseases may be severely crippling, but millions suffer quick and unsuspected deaths, and millions more suffer slow agony, uncertainty and equally untimely deaths.
>
> In the absence of accepted definitive views concerning the cause of the common degenerative diseases, speculation abounds. These are among the widely held views: 1. The degenerative diseases are mainly a natural consequence of aging and there is no

> way by which these processes can be prevented; 2. Heredity is a major factor in many of these conditions—such as coronary heart disease and diabetes—and again, one accepts the consequences fatalistically; 3. Many of these diseases are associated with emotional factors, such as tension of modern life and strained family relationships; 4. There is much discussion that autoimmune etiologies are the factor in arthritic diseases, and so on.
>
> A large and convincing body of scientific evidence, the subject of the chapters that follow, points in another direction entirely. The weight of this evidence indicates that the common degenerative diseases are largely due to nutritional factors, and do not require explanation in terms of such concepts as heredity, inevitability of aging, stress, etc. While acknowledged by only a small segment of the medical profession presently, recognition of the validity of the evidence upon which this viewpoint rests is gaining momentum.
>
> The evidence demonstrates that the cure for many of the degenerative diseases also has a nutritional basis: as the offending dietary factors are removed from the food regime, the symptoms of many of the degenerative diseases regress, often completely.

Pritikin's hypothesis was simple and profound: common foods in the diets of Westerners—especially in the United States—are overeaten in excess, causing a whole range of illnesses and premature death. Many of the medical world were skeptical of such talk, but some became interested. Pritikin collaborated in a study of dietary management for adult-onset diabetes. The Pritikin diet, which was low-fat, low-protein, and low-salt, was found to provide superior control of blood sugar than that regimen recommended at the time by the American Diabetes Association. He performed a study involving Veterans Administration (VA) patients with atherosclerotic heart disease and hypertension. The control group made no significant reduction in blood pressure or in diabetes. The experimental (Pritikin diet) VA group showed a marked decrease in blood pressure and cholesterol levels. The same was true for blood sugar levels and for other parameters of health that were monitored.

Longevity Center

With the results of two clinical studies to boost his confidence, Pritikin conceived the idea of establishing a rehabilitation center using diet and exercise as therapy. The center opened in January 1976 with the assistance of a physician who shared Pritikin's concepts regarding dietary intervention. Patients were often from out of town, and they stayed at a motel designated by Pritikin. For a twenty-eight-day period the group ate a Pritikin-specified diet, attended lectures, and exercised, while they were monitored by weekly physical examinations, various blood and treadmill tests, and chemical analyses of blood specimens. Smoking was prohibited. Graduation day was typically filled with tears of gratitude. Most of the people who went through the program believed that Pritikin had saved or substantially improved their lives. The vast majority of the people who came to the Longevity Center were seriously ill "medical failures," as they were termed by Pritikin.

Pritikin corresponded with Walter Kempner in 1976 and acknowledged that he was familiar with all that had been accomplished at Duke University.[20] The low-fat, low-protein, and low-salt dietary regimen that he prescribed for the West Coast "medical failures" was nearly identical, he noted, to that of the Duke program. After that initial introduction the two never established a personal relationship. From the prospective of several years following the death of each man, one sensed that each was busy with many patients to manage and had little time to derive a sense of satisfaction that their two revolutionary programs were similar.

The clinical improvement that Pritikin obtained for his patients was impressive. During the first year he could claim that of 218 certified hypertensives, 186 (85 percent) left, after twenty-eight days, with a normal blood pressure and no drug dependency. The average drop in cholesterol was 25 percent. Fifty to 80 percent of adult-onset diabetics left without requiring insulin or oral drugs. Word of such success spread and soon *60 Minutes* news teams appeared to make their appraisal. They were impressed, and the show that was put together in 1977 was a bombshell. Pritikin had been launched.

In 1978 Pritikin moved the Longevity Center to Santa Monica where a larger facility was available for the many patients who clamored for services. During the next several years twenty-five thousand medical cripples would seek care at the Pritikin Longevity Center.

Personal Health Problem

In 1965 routine blood testing showed that Pritikin had some abnormal values that suggested early-stage leukemia. Those laboratory results persisted and in 1976 it became apparent that Pritikin had chronic lymphocytic leukemia.

The leukemia was thought to be the result of radiation treatment he had received for a skin rash in 1955. Fortunately, the problem remained in abeyance and Pritikin was able to continue his work activities with the Longevity Center at a brisk pace. Only a few trusted friends knew of the leukemia, which did not cause physical hardship until late 1984. At that point progression was rapid. By February 1985 severe liver and kidney damage had occurred and dialysis had to be instituted. When his personal nurse and his wife had exited his room one evening for dinner, Pritikin cut his arteries at the elbow with a scalpel as a drastic alternative to hopeless life support. He immediately bled to death.

In the autopsy report, the pathologist noted: "Coronary arteries show minimal yellow discoloration of the intima [inner lining of the artery wall] but there are no plaques [cholesterol deposits] and the lumens are widely patent [open and smooth]." In his summary the pathologist concluded, "Absence of atherosclerosis, except for small fatty streaks, is unusual in a man of this age."

Respect and Acceptance

Before he died, some degree of respect and acceptance had been shown by the medical world to Pritikin. Studies were beginning to be published by medical institutions around the world that supported his views. Just two years after Pritikin's death, the *Journal of the American Medical Association* announced a study that showed regression of atherosclerosis in humans. The results followed a reduction in blood cholesterol that averaged 26 percent for the patient group, a drop similar to the one achieved at the Pritikin Longevity Center.

In 1966 Pritikin made the claim that coronary atherosclerosis could be reversed by lowering blood cholesterol. Twenty-one years later he had been vindicated.

Pritikin's Legacy

Pritikin had a keen awareness about many of the diet-induced maladies that affect people of the Western world. In his lectures he emphasized that gallstones and kidney stone are surely related to dietary improprieties. His interest extended far beyond atherosclerotic heart disease. Osteoporosis was recognized by him to be a problem of excessive dietary salt intake. And claudication (insufficient circulation to the legs) was a problem that could be relieved by the improved heart function that his low-fat, low-protein, and low-salt diet provided. He recognized that thirst was dependent on dietary salt intake.

Today, the Pritikin Longevity Center continues its operations in Florida under the direction of his son, Robert, who, like his father, has exhibited a lifelong commitment to helping people restore themselves.

NOTES

1. Kempner, W. Anoxemia of the kidney as a cause of uremic acidosis: inhibitory effect of low oxygen tension on the deamination of amino acids in kidney tissue. *American Journal of Physiology* 1938;**123**:117–118.

Kempner, W. Inhibitory effect of low oxygen tension on the deamination of amino acids in the kidney. *Journal of Biological Chemistry* 1938;**124**:229–235.

2. Kempner, W. Treatment of kidney disease and hypertensive vascular disease with rice diet. *JAMA* 1944;**125**:60.

3. Goldring, W and Chasis, H. *Hypertension and Hypertensive Disease*. New York: Commonwealth Fund, 1994.

4. Fishberg, AM. *Hypertension and Nephritis*. 4th ed. Philadelphia: Lea & Febiger, 1939.

5. Ornish, D et al. Can intensive lifestyle changes reverse coronary heart disease? Five-year follow-up of the Lifestyle Heart Trial. *JAMA* 1998;**280**:2001–2007.

6. Kempner, W. Compensation of renal metabolic dysfunction treatment of kidney disease and hypertensive vascular disease with Rice Diet III. *North Carolina Medical Journal* 1945;**6**:61–87, 117–161.

7. Kempner, W et al. Effect of rice diet on diabetes mellitus associated with vascular disease. *Postgraduate Medicine* 1958;**24**:359–371.

8. Stead, EA. Walter Kempner: a perspective. *Archives of Internal Medicine* 1974;**133**:756–757.

9. See Ornish, D. Stating and the sole of medicine. *American Journal of Cardiology* 2002;**89**:1286–1290, which concluded with the following message to physicians: "We can reclaim our time-honored roles of being physicians and healers by encouraging and supporting our patients

as they wrestle with the difficult challenges inherent in major diet and lifestyle change rather than merely being technicians who are following algorithms that tell us which pills to dispense and at what dosage. We can incorporate both the art and science of medicine back into our practices, addressing the psychosocial, emotional, and spiritual dimensions of our patients that motivate their behaviors. I think that nothing less than the soul of our profession is at stake, and it is time for us to reclaim it."

10. Ciba is a pharmaceutical company with headquarters in Zurich and New York.

11. *Durham News & Observer*. October 19, 1997.

12. Much of the Stefan George section was derived from Robert E. Norton. *Secret Germany: Stefan George and His Inner Circle*. Ithaca and London: Cornell University Press, 2002, 847 pages and from personal correspondence with Barbara Newborg, MD, Kempner's longtime associate.

13. Norton, Robert E. *Secret Germany: Stephan George and His Inner Circle*. Ithaca and London: Cornell University Press, 2002, p. 728.

14. Ibid., p. 736.

15. Ibid., p. 745.

16. *Durham News & Observer*. October 19, 1997.

17. See *Scientific Publications* by Walter Kempner, MD. Volume I *Studies in Cellular Physiology*. Newborg, B (ed.). Durham, NC: Gravity Press, 2002, 399 pages.

18. The material for the Nathan Pritikin section has been drawn in large part from a 1988 Rodale Press book by Tom Monte and Ilene Pritikin, Nathan's wife. Unfortunately the biography is out of print, but used copies are sometimes available through outlets on the Internet. They present an inspirational and fact-filled story of a man who did much to further the health revolution in America.

19. Leonard, JN and Hofer, JL and Pritikin, N. *Live Longer Now: The First One Hundred Years of Your Life: The 2100 Program.* New York: Grosset & Dunlap, 1974, 232 pages.

20. Personal correspondence, Barbara Newborg, MD.

CHAPTER 14

NOTES AND ASIDES (DIABETIC RETINOPATHY, MACULAR DEGENERATION, AND CROHN'S DISEASE)

In the past it would have been considered questionable taste to include personal experiences in a technical book of this sort. If for some valid reason that must be done, one technique has been to retreat to the anonymity of the third person. The author is purposely departing from that precedent and presents this section in the first person. This is because my interest in the subject of blood pressure, dietary electrolytes, fitness, and the like is more than academic. It is firsthand, personal, and intimate.

PROFESSIONAL BACKGROUND

My professional life has been that of a retinal physician/specialist since 1965. Undergraduate training was in chemical engineering at Atlanta's Georgia Institute of Technology. Medical training was across town at Emory University. Next was an ophthalmology residency and, finally, a retina fellowship at the Massachusetts Eye and Ear Infirmary and Boston's Schepens Eye Research Institute. In 1965, at age thirty-three, my wife and I, and our two young children at the time, made our way to Houston. I had accepted an opportunity within the vast medical complex that was developing south of the downtown area.

PRACTICE IN HOUSTON

During the two-year interval in Boston my duties were primarily those of a surgical assistant to specialists who cared for retinal detachment patients and, when time permitted, that of a clinical research physician. In Houston, I soon learned that a surgical practice took time to develop. Referral patients were more likely to have medical problems of the retina, such as diabetic retinopathy and macular degeneration.

Initially, then, my role was more that of a diagnostician and therapist and less that of a retinal surgeon. When interventional therapy was required, laser coagulation, a newly developed technique for that time, was used, at first with great caution but soon with increasing frequency as the potential for the therapy became apparent.

I accepted the challenge of managing medical retinal problems with enthusiasm. Laser intervention, I soon found, proved to be quite effective in controlling devastating bleeding problems within the retina. For some patients, though, the visual recovery left much to be desired. Was there something more, I wondered, that could be done?

The retinal practice soon became demanding. Diabetic retinopathy and macular degeneration cause a disproportionate amount of visual difficulty in the United States. Diabetic retinopathy is the leading cause of legal blindness in the twenty-to-sixty-five-year age group, while macular degeneration assumes that designation for the sixty-five and older age bracket.

In the evaluation of patients with retinal disease, blood pressure becomes a routine determination. And, as I soon noted, the readings for patients requiring specialized retina care were often elevated. Blood sugar and cholesterol levels were also of concern, so office-type laboratory equipment was obtained. For many of the diabetic retinopathy and macular degeneration patients, control of the basic parameters of one's health was abysmal.

As an ophthalmologist my role did not include the substitution of antihypertensive or diabetes-supportive medications for some other type of my own choosing. Dietary modification could be recommended, nevertheless. I was aware of the remarkable results being obtained by Dr. Walter Kempner at Duke University in the management of hypertensive cardiovascular/renal problems with a low-fat, high-carbohydrate, and sodium-restricted diet.[1] So I began providing dietary advice along with retinal care.

Kempner also prescribed his dietary regimen to diabetic patients with heart and renal failure. Remarkable improvement in the circulatory status of such patients was noted, and for many with diabetic retinopathy, resolution of the hemorrhages and exudates was observed, too.[2] Hypertensive hemorrhages involving the retina were also noted to clear.[3] Those extraordinary effects from dietary intervention had been reported before the era of retinal laser therapy.

As time went by, it became apparent that many of my patients were respecting my dietary recommendations (low-fat high-carbohydrate with no more than 750 mg Na per day). And, for those who did, blood pressure readings improved. For those with diabetes, blood sugar control was often better. Cardiac function improved. And along with the improvement in general health status, the diabetic retinopathy became easier to control. Most important, the visual outcome was better.

For those diabetic patients in whom retinal congestion (swelling) was an accompaniment to the blood vessel instability, the improvement exceeded, I felt, that which could be provided by laser therapy alone (figs. 1A and 1B). Fewer laser marks were necessary to achieve the desired result.

Most of Dr. Kempner's patients were admitted to the Duke University Hospital for supervised care. Following discharge they remained in Durham until he felt that the clinical improvement was sufficient for departure from the area. He motivated, threatened, and encouraged, and for many of his patients, adherence to the dietary regimen was maintained. The improved medical status that he and his associates obtained was nothing less than sensational.

In the 1950s and 1960s, medications for controlling heart failure and high blood pressure became available, and the popularity of the Kempner-type dietary regimen waned. But for my patients, the Kempner-type low-fat, high-carbohydrate, and sodium-restricted diet was a logical recommendation and a suitable adjunct to the care that they were receiving.

MACULAR DEGENERATION

Next to diabetic retinopathy, macular degeneration ranks second among the retinal problems that have required my attention. Patients of the latter category are of the older age group, sixty-five and up usually. Often they suffer from circulatory problems such as high blood pressure, coronary artery disease, and congestive heart failure. Salt usage, I have found, has been a consistent part of their dietary routine for much of their lives.

The clinical picture of macular degeneration varies over a wide spectrum, yet yellowish deposits within the central (the macular) retina are, usually, the earliest finding (fig. 2). These deposits, termed *drusen*, are composed of protein and lipid material. The retina has a dual blood supply. Drusen are thought to occur from the blood vessel layer behind the retina.

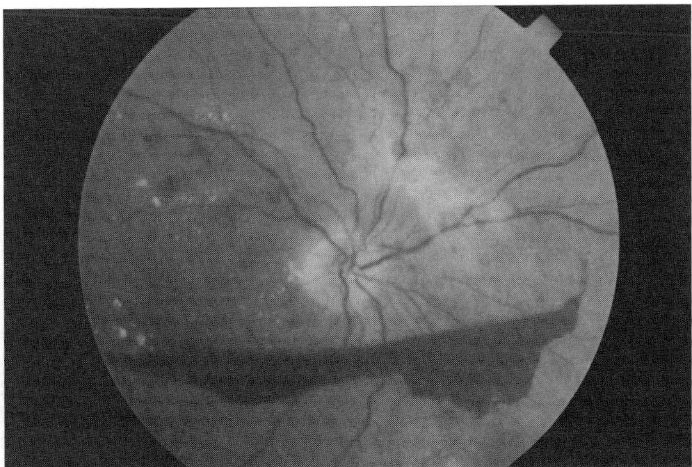

Fig. 1A. A thirty-eight-year-old male with a fourteen-year history of diabetes mellitus. Photo shows background and proliferative phase of diabetic retinopathy. A demanding low-fat, low-protein, and low-sodium dietary regimen was begun in June 1991.

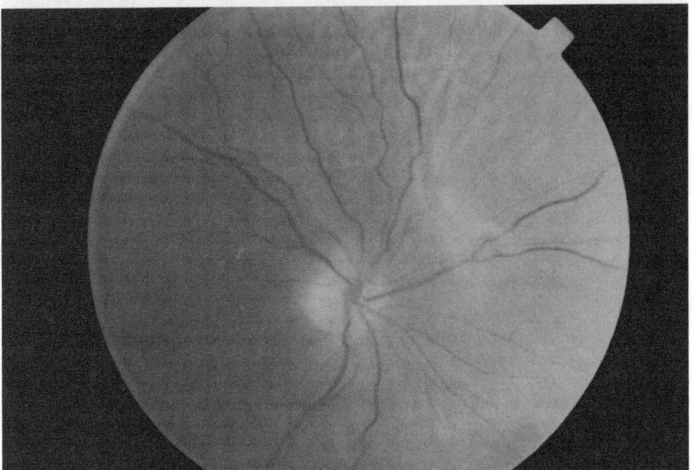

Fig. 1B. Resolution of diabetic retinopathy following adherence to a low-fat, low-protein, and low-sodium diet for three years. Photograph shows the same view for the right eye as figure 1A. The white exudates at left absorbed and the canoe-shaped hemorrhage cleared. For comparable photographs see Kempner, W et al. Effect of rice diet on diabetes mellitus associated with vascular disease. *Postgraduate Medicine* 1958;**24**: 359–371.

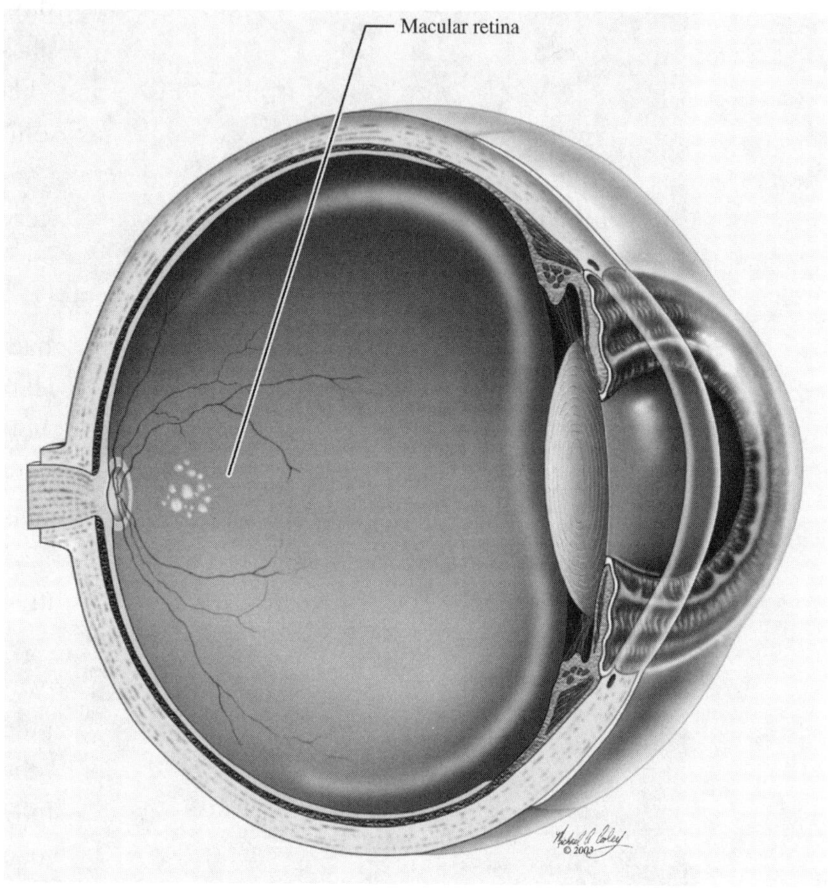

Fig. 2. Interior view of the left eye (artist's concept). The retina requires a dual blood supply—the inner vessels, as shown schematically in the diagram, and an outer membrane of vessels, not seen in such a view, that is applied to the posterior aspect of the retina. The protein and fat deposits that are depicted within the macular retina (arrow) are termed drusen. They develop between the retina and the outer network of blood vessels.

Early in my practice, I decided that a low-fat, high-carbohydrate, and sodium-restricted diet might be of value for macular degeneration patients, too. For those who would heed my advice (low-fat high-carbohydrate with no more than 500 mg Na per day) and make a persistent effort, partial resolution of the drusen has been observed on many occasions, a result which indicates that diet has a role in the development of drusen (figs. 3A and 3B). Resolution of drusen following dietary intervention compares to the clinical observations of Dr. Dean Ornish concerning coronary artery cholesterol deposits. He observed partial resolution of cholesterol plaques following adherence to a low-fat diet for two years.[4]

Confirmation that diet influences the progression of aged macular degeneration was recently established by researchers at Harvard University and the Massachusetts Eye and Ear Infirmary.[5] Volunteer subjects with early-stage macular degeneration were enrolled for a prospective study of 4.6 years duration. Participants with a body mass index of 25 or more were found to have a 2.3 times greater risk of developing advanced macular degeneration when compared with the normal-weight subjects.

Larger waist circumference (the so-called apple silhouette) was also found to be associated with a higher relative risk of developing advanced macular degeneration. Taken together, the results of the Harvard University/Massachusetts Eye and Ear Infirmary study suggest that the dietary effort that is applicable to maintaining good cardiovascular health extends to macular retina health, too.

A few months later (in 2004) further confirmation of a macular degeneration/dietary link appeared in the ophthalmological literature. Researchers found, in a prospective study of 77,562 female volunteers, a 36 percent decreased risk of neovascular ("wet-stage") macular degeneration when three or more servings of fruits are consumed daily.[6]

My retinal practice has now entered its thirty-ninth year, the entire period of which I have provided dietary counseling to patients with diabetic retinopathy and macular degeneration. I continue to be consistently impressed with the effect achieved by the strenuous

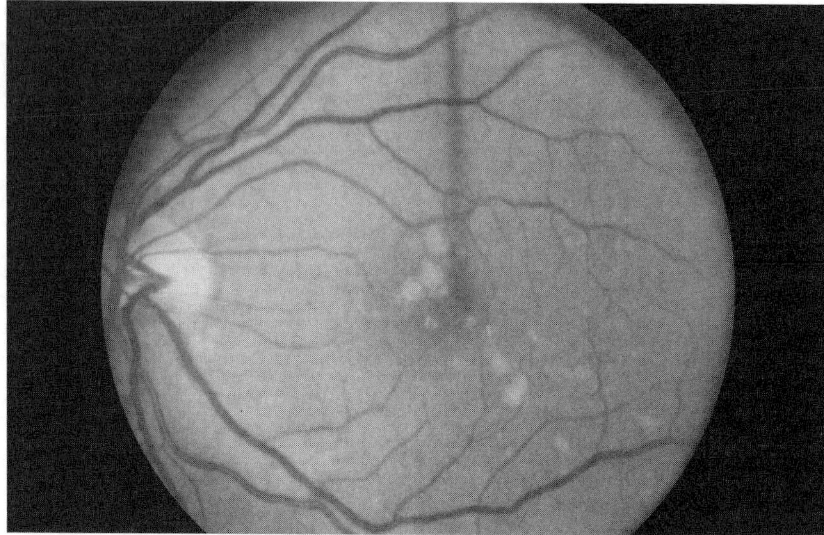

Fig. 3A. (Above) Photograph of nervehead and posterior retina for a sixty-two-year-old female. Soft drusen have formed deep within the macular retina of the left eye. BP 140/84. Visual acuity 20/25. The vertical line is a directional pointer within the camera.

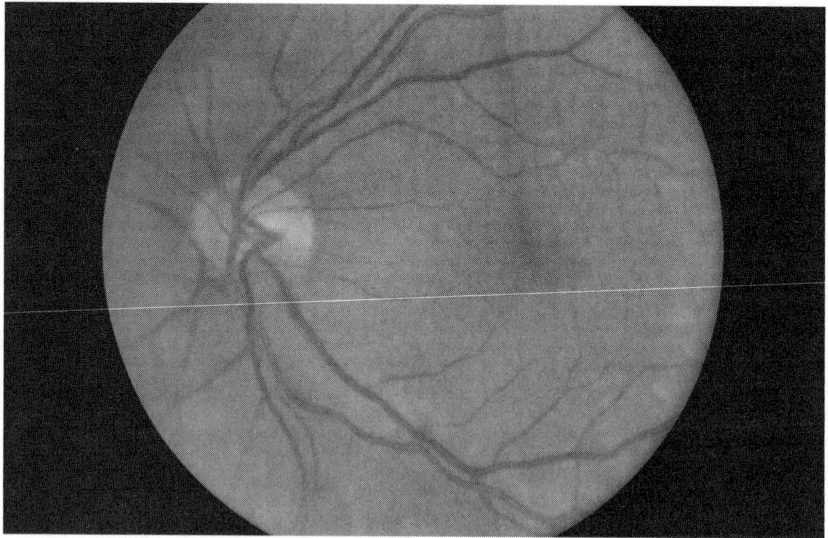

(Below) Thirty-three months later. A rigid low-fat and sodium-restricted diet was maintained during the interval. The soft drusen absorbed completely and the visual acuity improved to 20/20.

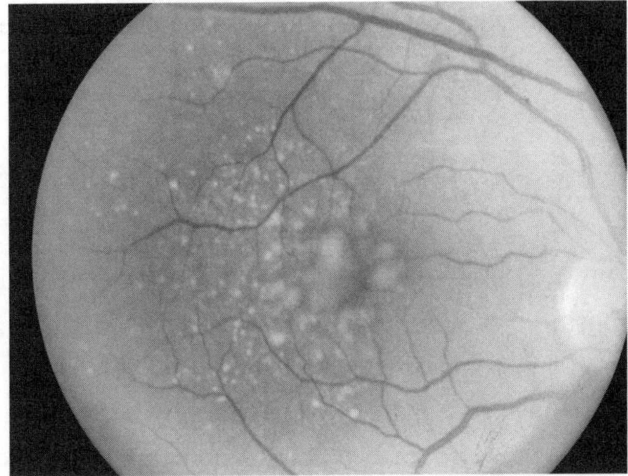

Fig. 3B. (Above) Photograph of nervehead and posterior retina for a sixty-eight-year-old female. Multiple soft drusen had formed deep within the macular and perimacular retina of the right eye. BP 142/86. Visual acuity 20/30.

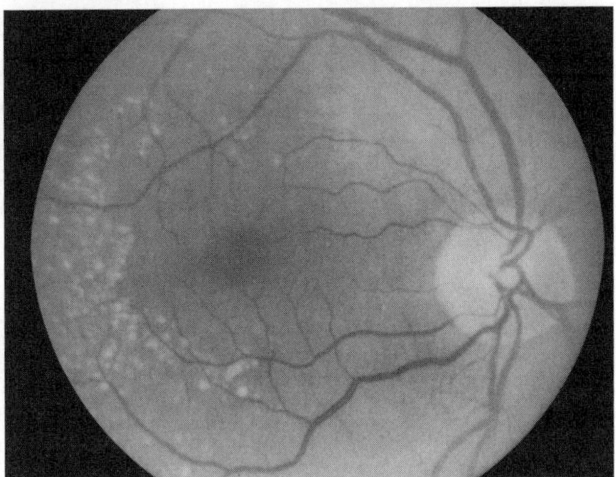

(Below) Thirty months later. Patient followed a rigid low-fat and 500 mg sodium-restricted diet. The soft drusen absorbed within the central macula (but not within the perimacular retina). The visual acuity for the right eye improved to 20/20.

The absorptin of drusen for this individual suggests that a 500 mg sodium diet reverses the abnormal egress of protein and fat molecules into the macular retina. The effect occurs, presumably, within a filtration membrane that separates the retina from a deeper layer of blood vessels, the so-called choroid.

effort of full compliance.[7] I do not prescribe vitamins, antioxidants, or dietary supplements. Improvement must come the old-fashioned way, following institution of rigorous dietary regimentation.

PERSONAL HEALTH EXPERIENCES

My own medical status was far removed from everyday thoughts during these initial practice years. But in 1972, at age forty, attention and concern began to include myself.

Because I had experienced a few headaches, monitoring of my blood pressure seemed a reasonable thing to do. And, to my surprise, the readings showed a mild degree of elevation for someone my age. In the early morning a pressure of 124/78 was usually obtained, but in the late afternoon, the systolic reading was higher, sometimes 132, 134, or 138. I considered such readings a poor start to my fifth decade of life and resolved that personal dietary patterns must be adjusted in a manner similar to that recommended to my patients.

The daily sodium intake was reduced to the 750 mg level. My wife, a pediatric pathologist, was cooperative. Our grocery lists were revised so that fresh foods were emphasized along with low-sodium cereals, breads, snacks, sauces, and the like. Within six weeks the systolic pressure decreased into the 124–128 range, and after a few months, the readings were likely to be 116 or so.

Today, in 2005, or thirty-one years later, I continue to maintain a 750 mg sodium-restricted diet. It's not that I count the milligrams daily, but it's that my diet is consistently limited to fresh foods and to those processed/packaged goods that are low in sodium. Blood pressure readings fluctuate between 104/66 and 126/74. There has been only one time during the past thirty years when it was higher. And that was ten years ago.

My weight had crept up to 165 pounds. I'm 5'11 1/2. With a

gain of six pounds, I found that systolic readings of 134 or so were again encountered.

I resolved to lose some weight. With a little effort, four pounds disappeared. And my blood pressure promptly decreased to its former level.

Another health parameter is pulse (heart) rate. Mine is often within the lower limit of normal, at 72 or so. I still manage my retinal practice and the required medical/surgical procedures six days a week. And I am left with plenty of energy for recreational activities and other pursuits (fig. 4).

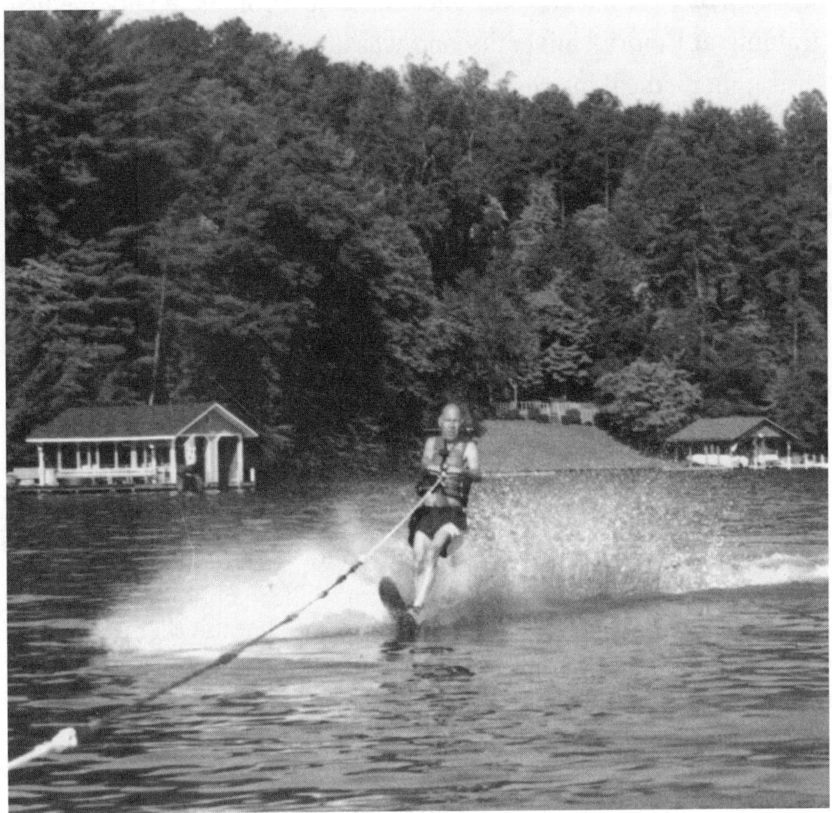

Fig 4. Lake Burton in northeast Georgia. The author, up from a submerged start and slalom skiing at age seventy-three.

CROHN'S DISEASE

Crohn's disease refers to inflammation within the small bowel characterized by recurrent attacks and remissions (fig. 5). The medical textbooks state that causative factors are assumed to be anxiety and nervous tension and maybe autoimmune response, which is to say: Crohn's disease, as far as textbook authors and editors are concerned, defies analysis. The textbooks also state that one million Americans, more or less, are afflicted with Crohn's.

In 1959, at age twenty-seven, I experienced the symptoms of Crohn's disease with a vengeance. I had just completed my medical training at Emory University and was approaching the midpoint of a straight medical internship program at downtown Atlanta's Grady Memorial Hospital.

Nowadays, my wife and I pass Grady Hospital each summer as we proceed along busy I-85 to our Lake Burton retreat in the Appalachian Mountains of northeast Georgia. Each time we pass, in a car that has been leased at Atlanta's Hartsfield airport following a ninety-minute flight from Houston, my thoughts recall that earlier struggle with Crohn's disease.

My first three months at Grady Hospital, in 1959, were somewhat rigorous—a work schedule on the medical floors that consisted of thirty-six hours on and twelve hours off. Next, came assignment to the pathology department, where my primary duty was that of an autopsy physician. The schedule was less demanding—twelve hours on and twelve hours off. On one memorable afternoon, during that latter interval, I developed persistent abdominal discomfort. By early evening the intensity of my symptoms had intensified, and the presumptive diagnosis of appendicitis was made by a couple of colleagues. Abdominal surgery was performed that evening.

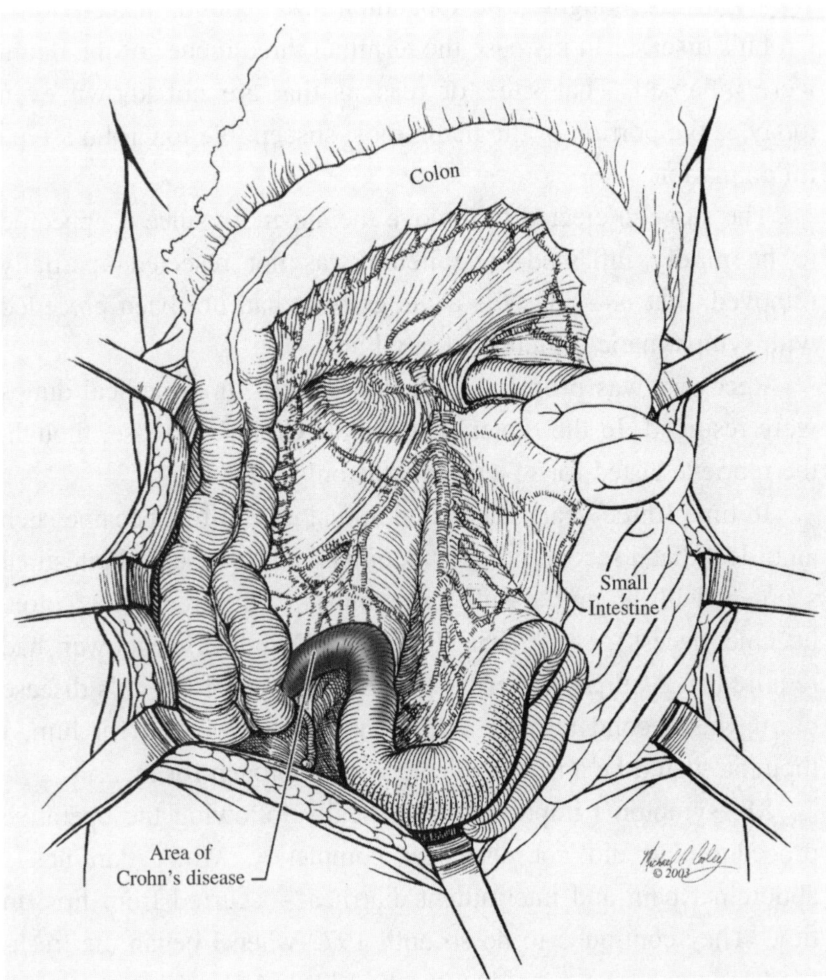

Fig. 5. Abdomen. Surgical view of the large (the so-called colon) and small (the jejunum and ileum) intestine. The small intestine has been reflected to reveal inflammation involving the terminal part of the ileum at the small intestine/large intestine junction. The ileum proximal to the Crohn's inflammation is dilated as a result of partial obstruction.

What was thought to be appendicitis was found, instead, to be Crohn's disease. In my case the terminal three inches of the ileum were inflamed. That site, for reasons that are not known even today, is the portion of the ileum most susceptible to Crohn's-type inflammation.

The surgeon elected to remove the appendix since it appeared to be mildly inflamed. The ileum was not resected—partially removed, that is—since the acute episode had not been preceded with symptomatic difficulty of any kind.

Recovery was prompt and within a short time medical duties were resumed. In the typical pattern for Crohn's disease, though, the reprieve lasted for several months only.

In time (three years later), abdominal discomfort became such an ordeal that a second procedure, bypass of the diseased intestinal segment with an end-to-side anastamosis to the transverse colon, became necessary. In 1956 President Dwight Eisenhower had required such surgery after he sustained a bout of Crohn's disease during his second term in office.[8] What had worked for him, I thought, would be a reasonable surgical approach for me.

My symptoms improved dramatically following the operative procedure but did not disappear completely. Minor flare-ups—abdominal pain and intermittent diarrhea—occurred from time to time. They continued to do so until 1972 when I began the fresh-food and low-sodium regimen for the 132–134 blood pressure readings. Shortly thereafter, my Crohn's disease symptoms disappeared, gradually at first and then completely. What a surprise! And what a sense of relief!

A low-fat, low-protein, and low-sodium diet reversed my Crohn's disease. More precisely, it was the salt restriction that had been responsible, I felt. A low-fat dietary regimen had been my dietary preference even before the onset of Crohn's disease.

DIET AND INTESTINAL DISEASE

In the early 1970s diet was first proposed as a contributing factor to the development of many gastrointestinal diseases. Hugh C. Trowell and Denis P. Burkitt, British physicians who practiced for many years in Uganda, documented in the medial literature that Africans have a low incidence of gastrointestinal diseases such as appendicitis,[9] Crohn's disease,[10] colitis,[11] diverticulitis,[12] duodenal ulcer,[13] colon cancer,[14] and constipation.[15] They postulated a protective effect for fiber-rich foods, which were the staple of the Ugandan diet at that time.[16] The bowel movement of the rural African natives, they noted, was bulky and soft, in contrast to the compacted stool of many Europeans and Americans. And the transient time was much less—a few hours instead of the two- to five-day typical passage for Europeans.

Other scientific papers regarding dietary fiber followed. And in short time, food manufacturers began including fiber-content information within the nutritional labels on their products. Much earlier in the twentieth century, J. H. Kellogg[17] had lectured and written on the contribution to health of whole cereal foods and had advocated the use of bran. Kellogg's views made little progress with the medical profession, however, as the leading American gastroenterologist of the time, W. C. Alvarez,[18] effectively counseled that man was a carnivore and should not eat extra roughage, which he condemned with great vigor.

Additional studies followed in midcentury, but the subject of dietary fiber was not widely discussed until Burkitt revived the subject in the late 1960s.[19] Studies subsequent to the 1970s have supported the contention that some amount of fiber is essential for normal intestinal function. The hypothesis that a generous fiber intake is necessary to prevent a variety of Western world ailments, including Crohn's disease, has not been proved, however.

TREATMENT FOR CROHN'S DISEASE

In the United States Crohn's disease is traditionally treated with corticosteroids, a hormonal anti-inflammatory medication. Clinical remission occurs in four to six weeks in 60 to 90 percent of patients.[20] About 15 percent of these who obtain remission on prednisone, the corticosteroid most commonly used, become medication dependent (defined as exacerbation of the ileitis within thirty days following discontinuation of the corticosteroid).

Two-thirds of those who remain in remission following discontinuation of the prednisone relapse within eighteen months. Crohn's disease is truly a chronic, relapsing, and remitting disease. Gastroenterologists in the United States consider treatment of Crohn's disease to be palliative rather than curative.[21]

In England, especially, and in continental Europe, to a lesser degree, physicians are more prone, in comparison to the United States, to advocate dietary modification for management of Crohn's disease.[22] One is inclined to think that the reports of Hugh Trowell and Denis Burkitt in the 1970s have been responsible for that choice in management.

Bacteria have never been identified as a cause for Crohn's disease. Neither have dietary antigens or autoantibodies (i.e., autoimmune mechanisms). So it seemed reasonable to physicians in England, and in Europe, too, that a dietary idiosyncrasy of some type or another could be responsible for the Crohn's disease, and if so, dietary modification should be a reasonable treatment approach.

Elemental Liquid Diet for Acute Episode of Crohn's Disease

The dietary regimen that has been used in England is a commercially prepared elemental mixture consisting of amino acids, carbohydrates, electrolytes, and vitamins. The two most commonly used pharmaceutical preparations are Flexical and Vivonex[23] (table 1). The caloric intake, which varies according to the amount consumed, is adjusted by the attending physician according to the needs of the patient. After the diagnosis of Crohn's disease has been established, the elemental mixture is drunk from a glass under professional supervision during the first few days of hospital care following which clinical improvement is usually sufficient for most patients to be discharged to their homes.

Following commencement of the elemental diet therapy, remission is achieved for 85 percent of patients with acute Crohn's disease, a percentage that compares favorably with the results

Table 1. Nutrient Content of Element Diets That Have Been Used in the Management of Crohn's Disease*

	Flexical† *Per 1000 calories*	*Vivonex‡* *Per 1000 calories*
Protein grams	32	50
Carbohydrate grams	138	175
Fat grams	38	12
Sodium	**510**	**670**
Potassium	950	800
Calcium	1600	670
Magnesium	200	110

* Vitamins not shown

†Bristol-Myers Squibb Item Code: OBI 9021 xx 07 HL

‡Novartis Nutrition Vivonex RTF

obtained by corticosteroid therapy. Some 23 percent of patients initially treated with an elemental diet subsequently require corticosteroid therapy for long-term maintenance, nevertheless.[24]

Of note is the low sodium intake with elemental diet therapy—500 to 1000 mg of sodium per day, depending on the amount consumed. I feel that the sodium limitation helps explain the clinical improvement obtained with Flexical and Vivonex. Sodium has long been used in enema preparations to cause bowel irritation and induce diarrhea. It only stands to reason that dietary sodium should be limited for patients who experience diarrhea and abdominal cramping from Crohn's disease.

After remission is obtained during the hospital stay with elemental diet therapy, the Crohn's disease patient resumes a normal routine at home. My thinking is that dietary sodium control must be continued over the long term. That's what has worked for me. It is reasonable to assume, finally, that other gastrointestinal diseases—gastric and duodenal ulcer, diverticulitis, irritable bowel syndrome, and ulcerative colitis come immediately to mind—could be ameliorated by the withdrawal from processed and fast-food items and the substitution of fresh and unsalted foods. As more experience with elemental dietary therapy is obtained, such an approach seems destined to assume a prime role in the management of gastrointestinal diseases of all types.

PATIENT FRUSTRATION

It has not been surprising to find that the personal frustrations brought on by Crohn's disease are making their way to the book publishers. One such account, *Controlling Crohn's Disease the Natural Way*, by Virginia Harper,[25] deserves recounting here. Hers is a mesmerizing tale of full-blown and unrelenting Crohn's disease; of a gastroenterologist's unwavering insistence on managing the bowel inflammation, despite a steady downhill clinical course, with prednisone, a corticosteroid, and Azulfidine, an antibiotic; and of ever-increasing side effects brought on by those medications.

In desperation Harper decided to place her fate with a therapeutic approach of her own choosing—a radical change in diet. She felt that the avoidance of processed foods was worth a try. At the next regularly scheduled appointment with her gastroenterologist, the aspects of that dietary menu—fresh vegetables, grains, fish, seeds, oils, and such—were presented, somewhat hesitantly. He was not impressed. Instead, he explained that methotrexate, a potent and dangerous immunosuppressant, was the only logical choice.

Harper followed her instincts, and, within a short period of time, following the switch to a macrobiotic (her term) diet, a miraculous subsidence in symptoms began. A little later, at the next appointment with the gastroenterologist, she again explained the basic aspects of the diet and the improved clinical status she was experiencing.

Her comments were met with an irate response. "The choice should be surgery," she was told. And as far as the macrobiotic regimen is concerned, "That diet is going to be too hard on you. You're going to hurt yourself."

"There's not one bit of scientific proof that a macrobiotic diet can be any good," Harper remembers him saying.

"How is it going to hurt me?" she asked.

"As your doctor, I can't allow it. You are in a very delicate condition and that crazy diet can only do you harm."

"I have already been doing it and it's helping me some. I want to give it more time," she said.

"You cannot remain on that macrobiotic diet. It's crazy and dangerous. I will not go on treating you if you do."

Harper relates that her physician's insolence hit her like a tornado. She left his office even more committed to avoid all processed foods.

The initial improvement continued as each week went by and ultimately the Crohn's disease was in remission. During the next twenty years (up to the time of the book's release), she remained symptom-free—no diarrhea, abdominal pain, indigestion, cramps, or fever.

GASTROENTEROLOGY PRACTICE IN THE UNITED STATES

Judging from the chatter at the inflammatory bowel disease Web sites and the tone of Virginia Harper's book, dissatisfaction with the treatment provided for Crohn's disease is increasing. That treatment in the United States is, without exception, medical and, if necessary, surgical. What is not provided is counseling regarding diet. The elemental diet therapy program of Great Britain is never offered as an option.

In March 2001 the American College of Gastroenterology (ACG) reissued practice guidelines for Crohn's disease management.[26] Only a short paragraph, shown below, was allotted to the subject of diet.

> Although elemental diets and possibly liquid polymeric diets[27] have demonstrated clinical benefits and reduce features of active Crohn's disease, the long-term course of disease is not altered, compliance is difficult in adults, and the cost is considerable. Elimination diets are not effective at preventing relapse after elemental diets.

That position statement by the ACG is misleading. The long-term course of dietary therapy has, simply put, not yet been studied. What is needed is a two- to five-year study comparing the efficacy of medical and dietary therapy. Is the ACG totally disinterested in such a project? Both patient compliance and cost of therapeutic management, the two other objectives raised by that organization, could be determined during such a trial.

What foods are responsible for Crohn's? That is the type of question that research investigators must consider. In the 1970s it was determined that Crohn's is a disease seen in the Western world and not in native populations. The implication that food processing is responsible for Crohn's is very strong.[28]

CONTROLLING CROHN'S DISEASE THE NATURAL WAY

Vicki Harper concluded her book with the following remarks. Few are capable of expressing it better.

> In this book, I have tried to show you how I overcame a very serious inflammatory bowel disorder, namely Crohn's disease, and how you can do it, too. Many so-called experts told me along the way that Crohn's is incurable and that what I was eating had nothing to do with it. The only way I could ever manage the illness successfully was with powerful drugs and surgery. Those who told me that had very authoritative credentials. They were highly educated. Yet, they were wrong.
>
> Looking back, I realize now that all I had was a belief in myself, a belief in those who tried to help me, and the willingness to trust my own experience. It is basic common sense. Food is definitely the first step, since it's our nourishment. And I mean real food—God-made food, not man-made food. The closer the food is to its natural state, its raw unrefined form, the higher its quality.
>
> In a society that expects everything fixed quickly without much personal input, being the steward of your own health becomes a major challenge. Society today has a "magic pill"

mentality. If it's not a pill, shot, or drink, we don't want to spend too much time thinking about it. We have luxurized saving time, but at what cost, if we are too sick to enjoy life?

NOTES

1. Kempner, W. Treatment of hypertensive vascular disease with rice diet. *American Journal of Medicine* 1948;**545**:117–161.

2. Kempner, W. Radical dietary treatment of hypertensive and arteriosclerotic vascular disease, heart and kidney disease, and vascular retinopathy. *GP* 1954;**9**:71–93.

Kempner, W et al. Effect of rice diet on diabetes mellitus associated with vascular disease. *Postgraduate Medicine* 1958;**23**:359–371.

3. Kempner, W. Treatment of heart and kidney disease and of hypertensive and arteriosclerotic vascular disease with the rice diet. *Annals of Internal Medicine* 1949;**35**:821–856.

Kempner, W and Newborg, B. Analysis of 177 cases of hypertensive vascular disease with papilledema, 126 patients treated with rice diet. *American Journal of Medicine* 1955;**19**:33–47.

4. Ornish, D et al. Intensive lifestyle changes for reversal of coronary heart disease. *JAMA* 1988;**280**:2001–2007.

5. Seddom, JM et al. Progression of age-related macular degeneration: association with body mass index, waist circumference, and waist-hip ratio. *Archives of Ophthalmology* 2003;**121(6)**:785–792.

6. Cho, E et al. Prospective study of intake of fruits, vegetables, vitamins, and carotenoids and risk of age-related maculopathy. *Archives of Ophthalmology* 2004;**122**:883–892.

7. Although my specialty is diseases and surgery of the retina and vitreous, I do encounter patients with other types of eye problems from time to time. And what I have found is that glaucoma patients also abuse dietary salt somewhat. I advise them to do otherwise and for those who are persuaded by my suggestion, a decrease in ocular pressure is often realized. In a recent exchange of communications with Trevor Beard,

MD, Senior Research Fellow, Menzies Research Institute, Hobart, Australia, I have learned that he, too, has obtained similar results with glaucoma patients. His book *Salt Matters: A Consumer Guide* (Melbourne: Lothian Books, 2004), contains much useful information regarding dietary sodium intake but is not available in international editions. For information, contact books@lothian.com.au.

8. Perret, G. *Eisenhower*. New York: Random House, 1999, pp. 534–535.

9. Burkitt, DP. The etiology of appendicitis. *British Journal of Surgery* 1971;**58**:695–699.

10. Trowell, H. *Non-Infective Disease in Africa*. London: Edward Arnold, 1960, pp. 216–219.

11. Trowell, H. Ulcerative colitis and Crohn's disease. In: *Refined Carbohydrate Food and Disease: Some Implications of Dietary Fibre*. Burkitt, DP and Trowell, HC. London: Academic Press, 1975, pp. 135–140.

12. Parnter, N and Burkitt, DP. Diverticular disease of the colon. In: *Refined Carbohydrate Food and Disease: Some Implications of Dietary Fibre*. Burkitt, DP and Trowell, HC. London: Academic Press, 1975, pp. 99–116.

Eastwood, MA and Eastwood, J and Ward, M. Epidemiology of bowel disease. In: *Fiber in Human Nutrition*. Spiller, GA and Amens, RJ (eds.). New York: Plenum, 1976, pp. 207–240.

13. Tovey, F. Duodenal ulcer and diet. In: *Refined Carbohydrate Foods and Disease: Some Implications of Dietary Fiber*. Burkitt, DP and Trowell, HC. London: Academic Press, 1975, pp. 299–310.

14. Burkitt, DP. Benign and malignant tumors of the large bowel. In: *Refined Carbohydrate Food and Disease: Some Implications of Dietary Fibre*. Burkitt, DP and Trowell, HC. London: Academic Press, 1975, pp. 117–133.

15. Burkitt, DP and Parnter, N. Gastrointestinal transit times; stool weights and consistency; intraluminal pressures. In: *Refined Carbohydrate Food and Disease: Some Implications of Dietary Fibre*. Burkitt, DP and Trowell, HC. London: Academic Press, 1975, pp 69–84.

16. Trowell, H. Refined carbohydrate foods and fiber. In: *Refined*

Carbohydrate Food and Disease: Some Implications of Dietary Fibre. Burkitt, DP and Trowell, HC. London: Academic Press, 1975, pp. 23–41.

17. Kellogg, JH. *The New Dietetics: A Guide to the Scientific Feeding in Health and Disease*. Battle Creek: Modern Medicine Publishing, 1923.

18. Alvarez, WC. Intestinal autotoxication. *Physiology Reviews* 1924;**4**:352–383.

Alvarez, WC. *An Introduction to Gastro-enterology*. London: Heinemann, 1931.

19. Burkitt, DP. Related disease—related cause? *The Lancet* 1969;**ii**:1229–1231.

20. Sanders, MD and Sarawicz, CM. Crohn's disease of the colon. In *Clinical Practice of Gastroenterology*, vol. 1 (ed.). Brandt, L. Philadelphia: Churchill Livingston, 1999, pp. 685–695.

21. Ibid.

22. Park, HR et al. Double blind controlled trial of elemental and polymeric diets as primary therapy in active Crohn's disease. *European Journal of Gastroenterology and Hepatology* 1991;**3**:483–490.

Raouf, AH et al. Enteral feeding as sole treatment for Crohn's disease: controlled trial of whole protein v amino acid based feed and a case study of dietary challenge. *Gut* 1991;**32**:702–707.

Gonzalez-Huix, F et al. Polymeric enteral diets as primary treatment of active Crohn's disease: a prospective steroid controlled trial. *Gut* 1993;**34**:778–782.

23. Sanderson, IR et al. Remission induced by an elemental diet in small bowel Crohn's disease. *Archives of Disease in Childhood* 1987;**61**:123–127.

Teahon, K et al. Ten years experience with an elemental diet in the management of Crohn's disease. *Gut* 1990;**31**:1133–1137.

24. Harper, V. *Controlling Crohn's Disease the Natural Way*. New York: Kensington Publishing Corp., 2002.

25. Ibid.

26. http://www.acg.gi.org/physicianforum/guides/index.html.

27. Polymeric is an expanded elemental-type liquid diet.

28. Elaine Gottschall, author of *Breaking the Vicious Cycle*, is

another who believes that one's dietary idiosyncrasies can be responsible for the development of inflammatory bowel disease. She advises withholding processed meats (hot dogs, cold cuts, and the like) and fast foods and emphasizes fruits and vegetables. Her advice seems sensible, indeed.

A contrary point of view is taken by the Crohn's and Colitis Foundation of America (CCFA), a fifty-thousand-member advocacy group. Its Web site (www.ccfa.org) material states: "There is no evidence that any particular foods cause or contribute to Crohn's disease or other types of inflammatory disease," a statement that avoids, for reasons not apparent, mention of the relatively good results that have been reported with elemental and polymeric diets. It is worth noting that the CCFA's activities are supported in large part by an array of pharmaceutical companies that produce medications for the management of inflammatory bowel disease. Unlike pharmaceuticals, fresh-food dietary therapy, which lacks a financial interest, has no advocate.

CHAPTER 15

HIGH BLOOD PRESSURE—DEVELOPING AN UNDERSTANDING

The effect that full commitment to a low-fat, sodium-restricted diet has on blood pressure is prompt. Consider the blood pressure plot obtained by the DASH Research Group during the 1997 trial[1] (fig. 1). Within two weeks the diet had reduced systolic pressure by 5.5 mm Hg, following which the readings were essentially unchanged during the remaining weeks of the trial. Kempner was the first to notice such dramatic results. He illustrated that effect in a 1948 report, with a blood pressure tracing for one of his patients, RL, a twenty-three-year-old male who achieved an extraordinary reduction in blood pressure within one month of rice-diet intervention[2] (fig. 2).

Pritikin counselors recently announced similar findings in *Circulation*,[3] the prestigious publication of the American Heart Association. The research volunteers were eleven obese men with hypertension, hypercholesteremia, and diabetes. Following three weeks of intensive dietary therapy, the men experienced (1) an average decrease in blood pressure from 162/100 to 138/82, (2) a 19 percent

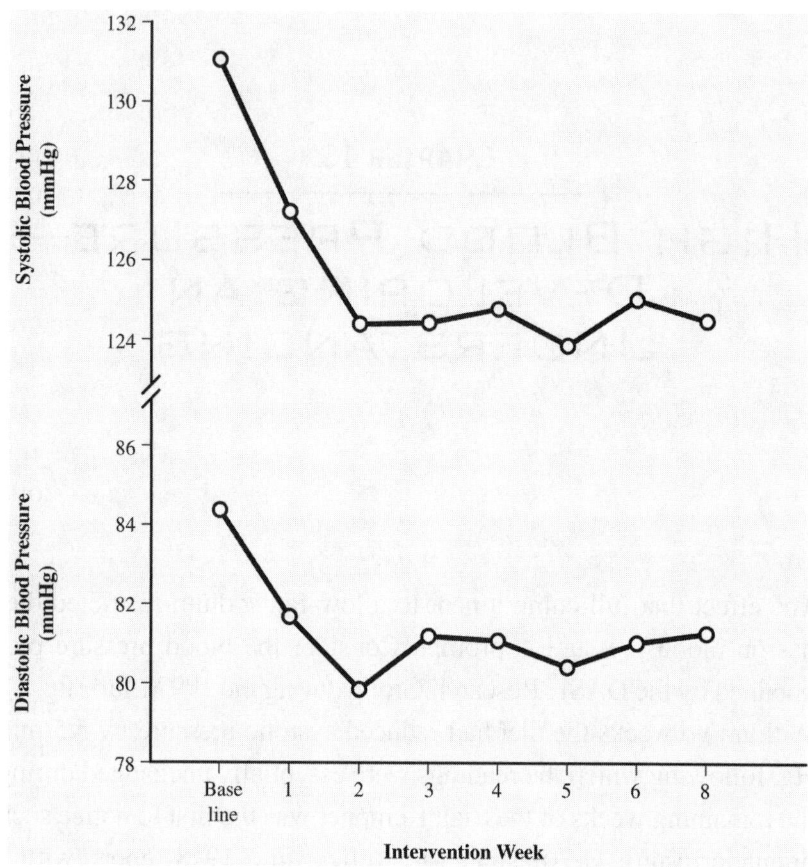

Fig. 1. Mean systolic and diastolic blood pressure at base line and during each intervention week for volunteer subjects (120 adults) who were placed on enhanced fruit/vegetable and low-fat diet (the 1997 DASH study). Improvement in blood pressure was realized during the first two weeks. (Reproduced with permission from Appel, LJ *New England Journal of Medicine* 1997;**336**:1117–1124. Copyright 1997 Massachusetts Medical Society)

decrease in cholesterol, and (3) a 46 percent plunge in the insulin requirement along with a 17 percent decrease in blood glucose. That improvement took place even though the men had only begun to shed weight. "You don't have to wait till you've lost a lot of weight to get major reductions in heart disease risk," stated Dr. James

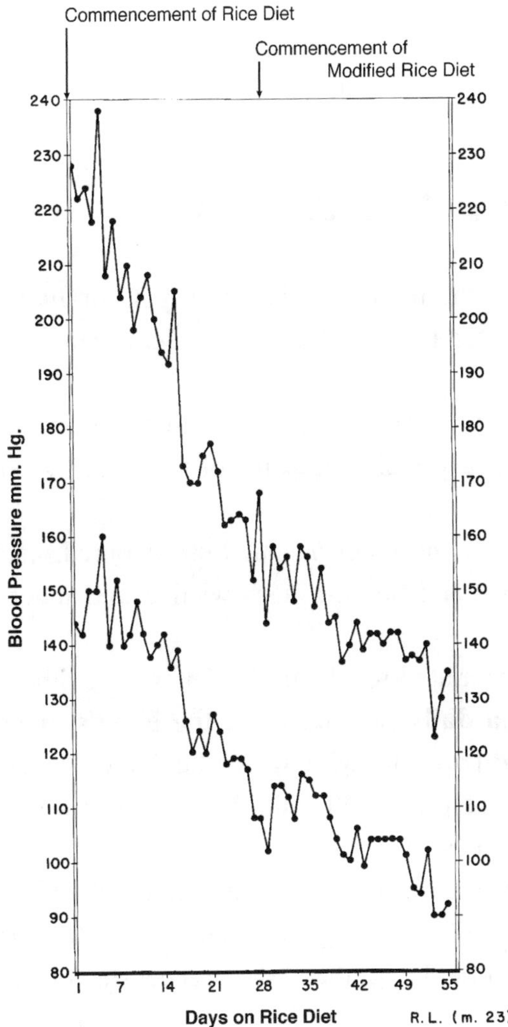

Barnard, lead author and UCLA professor of physiological science. "Fortunately, you can mitigate high blood pressure and the risk of heart attack while, or even before, you shed excess pounds."

A dramatic improvement in blood pressure and general sense of well-being has been my experience with patients who make a full commitment to dietary intervention. Of course, much of the time the commitment comes gradually, even grudgingly, and sometimes not at all. But when the dietary adherence

Fig. 2. This twenty-three-year-old patient had hypertensive vascular disease of three years' duration. Cholesterol was 340 and kidney function was impaired. Rice/fruit diet was started on December 18, 1945, and was followed strictly. By March 1946 kidney function had improved and the cholesterol level was 173. (Reprinted from Kempner, W. Treatment of Hypertensive Vascular Disease with Rice Diet, *American Journal of Medicine* 1948;**4**:545–577, copyright 1948 with permission from Excerpta Medica, Inc.)

is full and steadfast, results come right away. On such occasions, an astounding passage in the Old Testament involving the youthful Daniel and his companions comes to mind.[4]

FROM THE BOOK OF DANIEL, CHAPTER 1

1. In the third year of the reign of Jehoiakim King of Judah came Nebuchadnezzar King of Babylon to Jerusalem and besieged it.
3. And the King ordered Ashpenaz, his chief, to bring certain of the children of Israel, including some of the King's seed and of the nobles,
4. children in whom was no blemish, but well favoured, and skillful in all wisdom, and cunning in knowledge, and understanding science.
5. And the King appropriated for them (Daniel and the others that were chosen) **a daily portion from the King's meat and provision, and from the wine which he drank** and so appointed that they be provided for three years, after which they were to enter the King's personal service.
8. But Daniel decided in his heart that **he would not defile himself** with the portion of the King's meat and provision, nor with the wine which he drank; therefore he requested of the commander of the official that he might not defile himself.
12. "Please test you me and Hananiah, Mishael, and Azariah (son of Judah) for ten days, and let us be given **vegetables to eat and water to drink**."
13. "Then let our appearance be observed in your presence, and the appearance of the youths who are eating the King's choice food; and deal with your servants according to what you see."

14. So he listened to them in this matter and tested them for ten days.
15. And at the ends of ten days their appearance seemed better and they were fatter than all the youth who had been eating the King's choice food.
16. So the overseer continued to withhold the choice food and wine, and kept giving them the **vegetables**.
20. In every matter of wisdom and understanding about which the King questioned them (Daniel and his companions), he found them ten times better than all the magicians and enchanters in his whole kingdom.

As the 1997 DASH trial, the Kempner reports of many years ago, the *Circulation* report from the Pritikin program, and the biblical story of Daniel and his companions indicate, full dietary compliance can have a prompt effect on blood pressure and one's sense of well-being. To understand how the turnabout can occur so abruptly, consideration of the blood dynamics responsible for hypertension provides some insight.

Blood Pressure Dynamics

Blood pressure varies directly with *cardiac output*[5] (the amount of blood pumped each minute by the heart) and the *resistance to flow*. Resistance, in turn is the product of *blood viscosity* (fluidity) and the *hindrance* imposed by the blood vessels.

Cardiac output remains reasonably steady during one's lifetime, or until a problem with the contractibility of the heart muscle develops. Flow studies of patients with high blood pressure have shown that cardiac output has remained unchanged, essentially, during the course of the disease. Therefore, it is not cardiac output but the resistance to blood flow that is the dynamic aspect of established hypertension.

Hindrance represents the contribution of blood vessel geometry to resistance (narrowing and constriction). A long-term effect of hypertension is arteriolar wall thickening (arteriosclerosis, narrowing). Constriction is the result of smooth muscle contraction within the wall of the arterioles.

A significant correlation between *blood viscosity* and blood pressure has been demonstrated in patients with hypertension[6] (fig. 3). Blood viscosity is increased in patients with hypertension even in the early or borderline phase.

Flow Properties of Blood: Blood is a complex aqueous system consisting principally of plasma proteins, electrolytes, and three formed elements—red cells, white cells, and platelets. Of the proteins, it is albumin that appears to play the key role in maintaining blood stability, that is, the suspension of the formed elements, discretely and without clumping.

In health, the formed elements of blood remain discrete. The cells bear a negative charge that creates mutual repulsion. (Objects of similar charge repel each other; objects of opposite charge attract.) That the elements within blood bear a negative charge was shown, many years ago, by applying a current in a cataphoresis chamber; red blood cells (RBCs) moved promptly to the anode (the positive electrode).

It is essential that RBCs do not adhere to each other, or to the walls of the arterioles and the capillaries. In the capillary bed the RBCs release oxygen to the immediately adjacent tissues, throughout the entire body, and absorb bicarbonate, a waste product. The bicarbonate is absorbed into the serum and transported to the capillaries within the lungs for release as carbon dioxide during expiration. Good efficiency requires that the entire surface of an RBC contribute to the exchange that occurs within the capillaries.

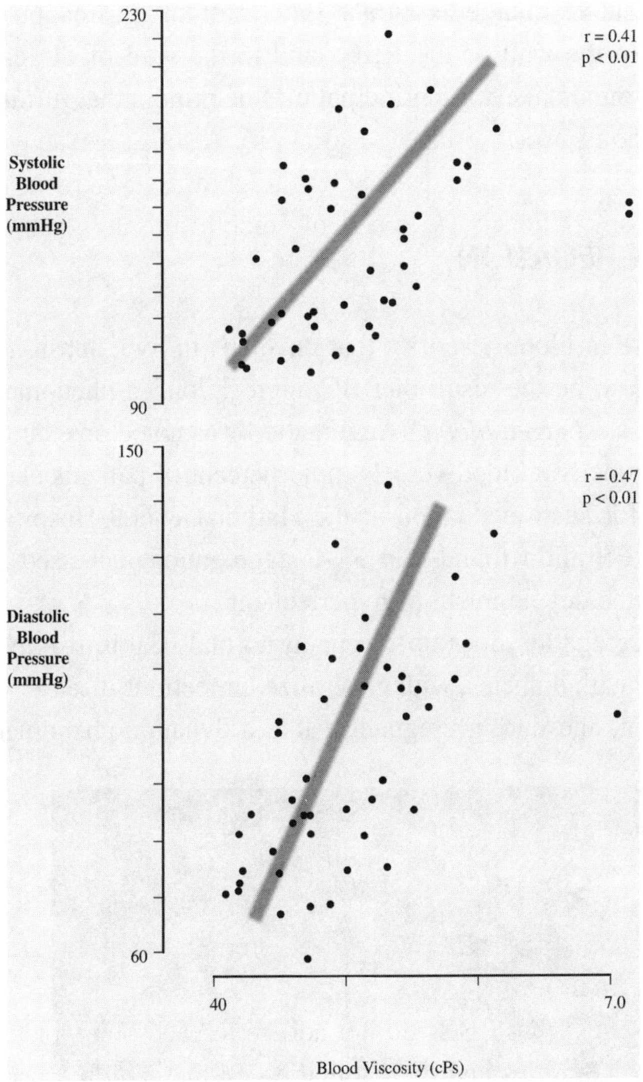

Fig. 3. Correlation between blood pressure and blood viscosity in normal controls and patients with high blood pressure. The plot lines define the trend for systolic and diastolic blood pressure.[7] (Reproduced with permission from Letcher, RL et al. *American Journal of Medicine* 1981;**70**:1195–1202) An increase in viscosity can be due to an elevation of any one of the blood pressure viscosity determinants or their combination. Of those determinants, red blood cell aggregability has the greatest effect.

The negative charge is surely the result of plasma protein adherence to the wall of the RBCs and to the wall of the capillaries. Albumin is likely the principal plasma protein that furnishes that protection.

RBC AGGREGATION

The increase in blood viscosity that develops in hypertension has been shown to be the result of RBC aggregation,[8] a phenomenon also known as *sludged blood*.[9] Aggregation was noted on examination of conjunctival blood vessels in 83 percent of patients chosen at random for such evaluation at the Harbor General Hospital in 1949.[10] A. Petralido found that RBC aggregation increased precisely with the development of hypertension.

RBC aggregation does not occur in normal health. It is noted particularly with diabetes, with generalized infectious disease, with hypertension, and during pregnancy. It is a dynamic phenomenon

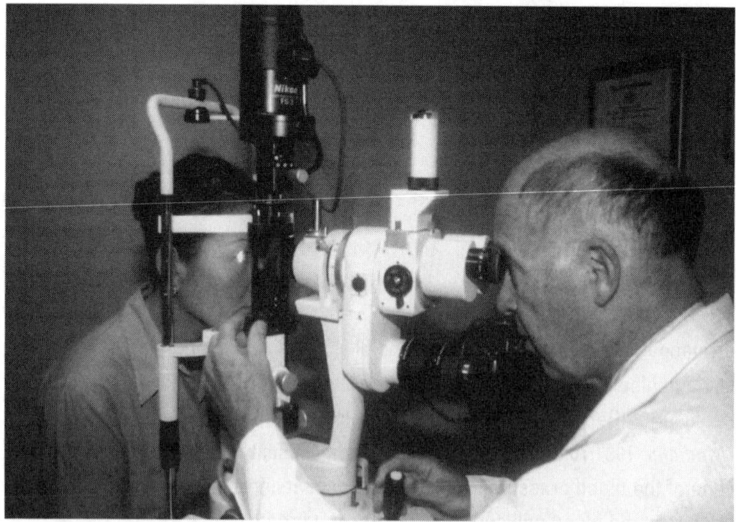

Fig. 4. Examination technique for viewing RBC aggregation.

and the one that is capable of explaining the abrupt decrease in blood pressure that followed full dietary compliance for the DASH Research Group, for Pritikin physicians, and for Dr. Kempner. RBC aggregation is capable of both rapid onset and rapid reversal.

Clinical Appearance

RBC aggregation can be studied in the conjunctiva of the eye with a suitably adapted microscope[11] (fig. 4). The *conjunctiva* is a thin, transparent membrane covering the white portion (the sclera, or outer tunic) of the eyeball.

For examination of the flow characteristics within the conjunctival blood vessels, a magnification of 60X is required. For research physicians intent on studying the phenomenon of RBC aggregation, microscopes have been fabricated to specification. The ophthalmologist has the best opportunity to perform the task with equipment already available: the slitlamp microscope. Even so, the objective and the eyepiece must be custom-ordered in order to meet the necessary specification of 60X. The currently available ophthalmological slitlamps with a maximum magnification of 30X are generally unsuitable.

For the past twenty years I have had two slitlamps that meet object magnification for aggregation evaluation. Those observations confirm that many—perhaps 85 percent of adults—demonstrate the aggregation phenomenon on a sliding scale of severity. I designate the variability in degree as follows (table 1).

Table 1. Grade and Degree for Intravascular Coagulation

Numerical Grade	*Aggregation*
0	absent
1	slight
2	moderate
3	considerable
4	heavy

In health most capillaries are substantially filled with discrete cells. The flow within capillaries is continuous and uniform. Aggregation is absent. The earliest indication of aggregation is evidence of "comets." A *comet* is a clump of

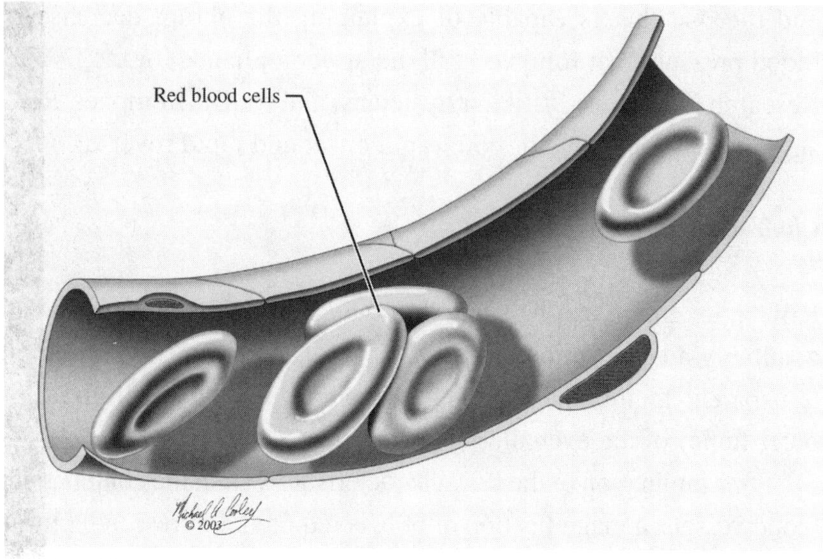

Fig. 5. Comets. A *comet* results when a capillary is filled primarily with clear plasma, instead of being filled uniformly with erythrocytes and other blood cells. Red cells will then dart singly or in small groups through the capillary, giving the impression of "shooting stars" or comets.

two to four cells that dart through the capillary with a space of clear plasma in between (fig. 5). Many cells remain discrete. That stage of slight aggregation is followed by more moderate clumping. The physical appearance of the blood flow becomes "granular." Next, the aggregation is more pronounced and stasis, or slowing, is noticeable in many of the smaller capillaries.

Sometimes the flow in a capillary under examination periodically comes to a faltering halt, reverses, then flows again into sluggish action. In the heavy stage (fig. 6) clumping is found in the arterioles and the venules, but it is often not evident in the smaller capillaries, where the small diameter permits red cells to traverse in single file only. With clumping, each cluster of cells is separated from its adjacent group by a "cylinder" of clear plasma.

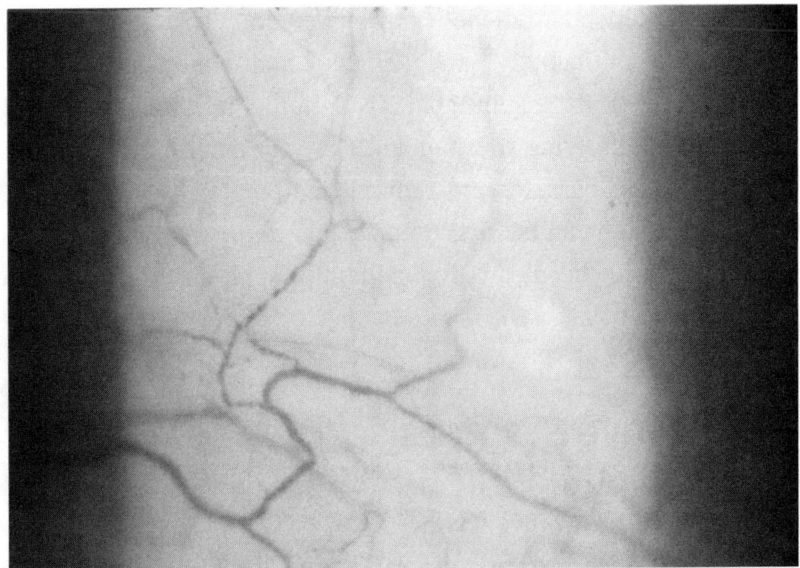

Fig. 6. Clumping. *Clumping* refers to RBC aggregation in individual groups of ten to one hundred. Clumps can be found in arterioles and venules. They are not evident in capillaries, the small diameter of which permits red blood cells to transverse in single file only.

During examination of the retina, the effect of RBC aggregation becomes particularly apparent in the capillary system of insulin-dependent diabetic patients who are developing proliferative (new blood vessel growth) retinopathy. These young and middle-age individuals often abuse the use of dietary salt, sometimes to an outrageous degree.

The RBC sludging slows the flow rate within the capillary system of the retina and, as an extension of that process, some of the smallest capillaries become obstructed. Eventually, the capillary segment collapses into a nonfunctioning threadlike strand.

Retinal circulation photography for these individuals often reveals multiple foci of nonfilling (fig. 7). The retina in those small areas, deprived of oxygen for cellular metabolism, becomes nonfunctional.

Insulin-dependent diabetics often develop circulation problems at other sites in the body—the toes, feet, and kidney, for instance—and one can safely assume that RBC clumping with capillary closure is the underlying mechanism. Care for such individuals must be directed, in part, toward reduction of the RBC clumping, the degree of which can be measured by laboratory analysis of a blood specimen. And the means for achieving such an effect is dietary electrolyte control.

SPECULATIVE HYPOTHESIS TO ACCOUNT FOR RBC AGGREGATION

My clinical observations have led me to the belief that the electrolyte imbalance of the modern diet is responsible to a considerable degree, if not entirely, for the RBC aggregation that occurs in hypertension. It is reasonable to assume that our kidneys were not designed to operate routinely at an overload greater than 200 to 500 percent. This would place the desirable limit of daily sodium intake at 500 to 1000 mgm. The chain of events is like this, I suspect: Sodium excess in conjunction with potassium, magnesium, and calcium deficiency alters not insignificantly the electrolytic charge for an RBC which, in turn, decreases the repulsive effect that the cells manifest for each other. Alternately, the electrolytic milieu within plasma is altered by the present-day topsy-turvy dietary electrolyte imbalance so that, in turn, the RBC repulsive force is diminished. Probably both the RBC cellular membrane and the plasma milieu are affected by electrolytic dietary imbalance.

The concept of repulsion for a colloid system (a fluid system with suspended particles), whether it be organic, such as blood, or inorganic, such as an industrial water treatment basin, depends on the force and the distance over which the RBCs, in the organic

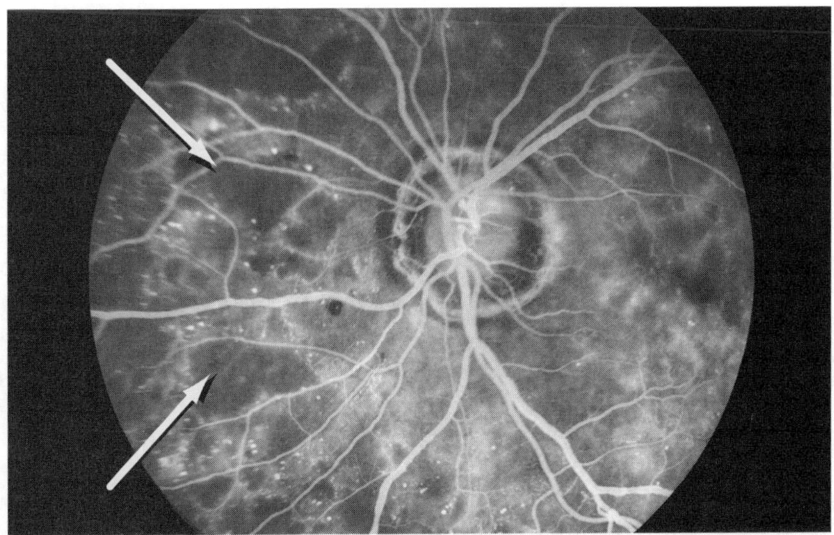

Fig. 7. Retinal circulation photograph for a thirty-one-year-old diabetic patient. In the dark sectors (arrows) the dye has failed to perfuse the capillary system. The nonfilling is the result of capillary obstruction secondary to RBC clumping. Such nutrient-deficient sectors are responsible for the dangerous phase of blood vessel proliferation (neovascularization) on the inner surface of the retina.

system, or particles, in the industrial water system, can repel each other and, by doing so, oppose aggregation. The negative surface of an RBC or the particle in a water treatment basin attracts a surrounding layer of positive electrolytes that may originate from the bulk of the suspending liquid or from the colloidal cell/particle itself (fig. 8). The oppositely charged electrolytes, or counter-ions, are drawn to the cell/particles by electrostatic attraction. If the negative charge is large, some counter-ions will stick to the surface. This layer partially neutralizes the charge and electrostatic attraction of the cells/particles. Other positive rows remain close to the surface but do not become attached.[12]

The attraction of the cell/particle is greatest, of course, close to itself, both because of the distance involved and also because the counter-ions near it impose their positive charge and thus shield those counter-ions farther away. Hence, the neutralizing counter-ions are most concentrated near the cell/particle and become gradually negligible farther away. Similarly, negative electrolytes tend to be repelled from the immediate vicinity of the cell/particle.

Zeta Potential is related to the force and distance over which the cells/particles can repel each other and prevent aggregation. It is the potential at the surface separating the immobile part of the double layer from the diffuse part.

When a liquid containing such charged particles is placed in an electric field, the negative particles are attracted to the positive electrode and the counter-ions to the negative. This attraction increases with the charge of the particle. Friction between the cell/particle and the surrounding liquid containing the diffuse double layers slows down the resulting motion toward the electrode—the greater the extent of the double layer, the lower the resistance. Therefore, particle velocity in a given field increases with both density and extent of the double layer, which are measured by the Zeta Potential. Hence, the velocity of a colloidal cell/particle in an electric field is proportional to that field (volts/cm) and to the Zeta Potential of the particle.

CROSSMATCH STUDIES

Hunter Little, a retina specialist, studied RBC aggregation in diabetic patients.[13] In an attempt to determine whether the decrease in electronegative potential (the decrease in Zeta Potential) was at the surface of the RBCs or in the plasma, crossmatch studies were performed between diabetic and nondiabetic subjects of the same blood type. When RBCs from a nondiabetic were combined with plasma of a diabetic with retinal vascular disease (diabetic retinopathy), the

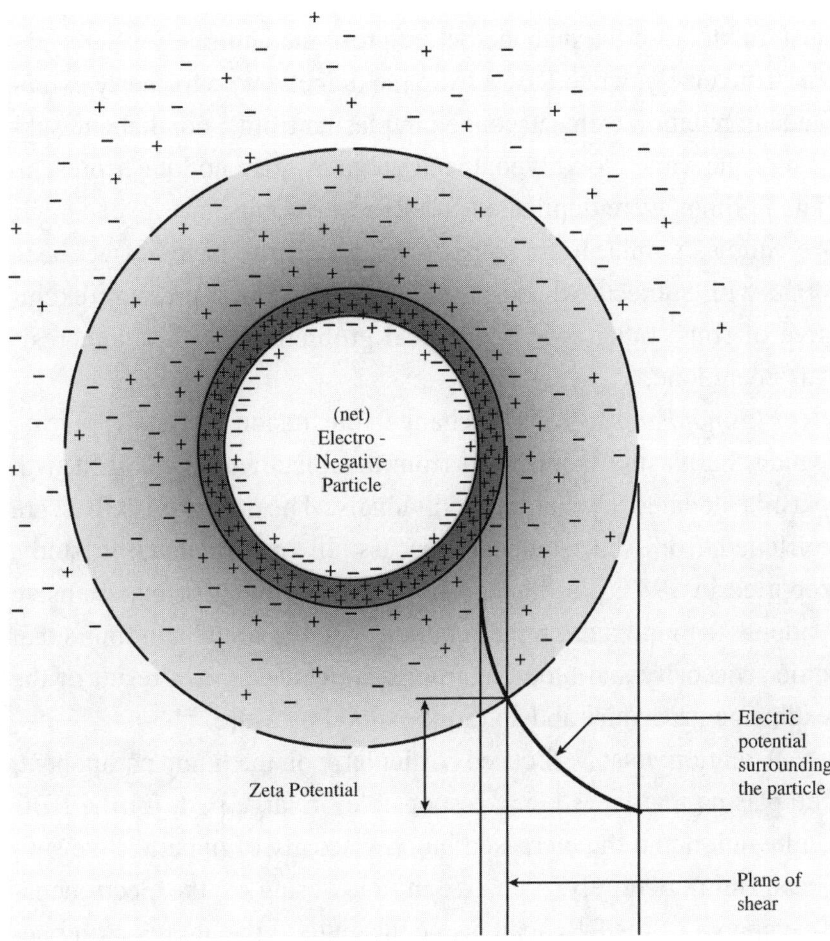

Fig. 8. Conventional concepts of Zeta Potential. (Reproduced from Riddick, TM *Control of Colloid Stability through Zeta Potential,* Pennsylvania: Livingston Publishing, 1968.) The diagram suffers from being planar rather than three-dimensional and from the inability of the draftsman to adequately picture the number and relative density of ions surrounding the particle.

RBCs from the normal subject clumped in a manner that had been seen in blood of the diabetic before cross-matching.

Conversely, when RBCs from the diabetic who formerly exhibited aggregation were suspended in plasma from a nondiabetic subject of the same blood type, the aggregates were no longer present. The findings were duplicated for several patients.

Studies similar to those performed by Little have not yet been done with subjects whose problem is high blood pressure exclusive of some other type of medical problem. But plasmapheresis has been done.

Plasmapheresis is an exchange transfusion technique during which the plasma is removed from a subject and exchanged with plasma donated by normal individuals. The subject's RBCs are excluded from the exchange process. In one challenging study, reported in 1983, plasmapheresis was performed for hypertensive patients with impaired renal function. The research team found that blood viscosity and blood aggregation decreases as a result of the exchange procedure and so did the blood pressure.[14]

Attention must be focused particularly on the liquid component, the plasma that is, as being responsible, in large part, for the RBC aggregation and the increased blood viscosity of hypertensive subjects. But not entirely. A change in (a lowering of) the electronegative charge of the RBC can also contribute to the aggregation phenomena. Research studies of patients with high blood pressure have demonstrated an increased sodium concentration within RBCs[15] that, in turn, decreases the repulsive force (and increases the tendency for RBC sludging).

High Blood Pressure: Prevention and Control of RBC Aggregation by Dietary Modification

The management of high blood pressure must include the elimination of basic causes. Control measures, such as medications, should be considered, in the best of circumstances, simply as a temporary expedient until dietary measures take effect. Those requiring high blood pressure care should be apprised of the blood sludging that develops as a result of sodium excess and potassium, magnesium, and calcium deficiency in the diet. With a proper balance of electrolytes, as provided by the 2001 DASH low-sodium regimen, RBC aggregation can be reduced and high blood pressure can be brought under control. I have observed such a sequence of events for those who make a full commitment to eat right—electrolyte.

Notes

1. Appel, LJ et al. A clinical trial of the effects of dietary patterns on blood pressure. *New England Journal of Medicine* 1997;**336**:1117–1124.

2. Kempner, W. Treatment of hypertensive vascular disease with rice diet. *American Journal of Medicine* 1948;**4**:545–577.

3. Roberts, CK et al. Effect of diet and exercise intervention on blood pressure, insulin, oxidative stress, and nitric oxide availability. *Circulation* 2002;**106**:2530–2532.

4. Daniel 1:1–20.

5. Cardiac output is the quantity of blood pumped into the aorta each minute by the heart. For a young, healthy, adult man, the resting cardiac output averages 5.6 liters (about 5.9 quarts) per minute. For women, this value is 10 to 20 percent less. The average cardiac output for adults is often stated to be 5 liters per minute.

With exercise, cardiac output increases because heart ratio increases. With increasing age, cardiac output decreases—by 20 percent or so at age eighty, because of both a decrease in heart rate and stroke volume (the amount of blood pumped into the aorta with each contraction of the heart).

6. Letcher, RL et al. Direct relationship between blood pressure and blood viscosity in normal and hypertensive subjects: role of fibrinogen and concentration. *American Journal of Medicine* 1981;**70**:1195–1202.

7. The slope of trend line is steeper for the diastolic pressure than it is for the systolic.

Physicians use the term *pulse pressure* to describe the difference between the systolic and diastolic readings. A person with a blood pressure of 120/80 has a pulse pressure of 120 minus 80, or 40.

In young adults an elevation in blood pressure is often associated with a narrowing of the pulse pressure. In diabetic patients, for instance, the examiner often finds the blood pressure to be 134/88 (pulse pressure of 36) or thereabouts. Diabetic patients consistently show RBC aggregability, which affects the diastolic pressure to a greater degree than the systolic.

In adults of advanced age, the opposite is true. Pulse pressure becomes widened. For instance, the examiner might find the blood pressure for an older adult to be 144/86 (pulse pressure of 54) or a similar combination thereof. The widening is due to thickening and narrowing of the arterioles that develops as a result of long-standing hypertension.

8. Petralito, A and Malatino, LS and Fione, CE. Erythrocyte aggregation in different stages of arterial hypertension. *Thrombosis and Haemostasis* 1985;**54**:555.

Zannad, F et al. Haemorheological abnormalities in arterial hypertension and their relation to cardiac hypertrophy. *Journal of Hypertension* 1988;**6**:293–297.

9. Kniseley, MH et al. Sludged blood. *Science* 1947;**106**:431.

10. Bellis, CJ and Snow, HL. Sludged blood: the electrokinetic factor involved. *Annals of Western Medicine and Surgery* 1950;**4**:223–226.

11. Ditzel, J. The nature of the intravascular erythrocyte aggregation in diseases with particular reference to diabetes mellitus. *Acta Medica Scandinavica* 1955;**5**:371–378.

Little, H. The role of abnormal hemorrheodynamics in the pathogenesis of diabetic retinopathy. *Transactions of the American Ophthalmological Society* 1976;**LXXIV**:573–632.

12. Riddick, TM. *Control of Colloid Stability through Zeta Potential.* Wynnewood, Pennsylvania: Livingston Publishing Company, 1968, p. 198.

13. Ditzel, J. The nature of the intravascular erythrocyte aggregation in diseases with particular reference to diabetes mellitus. *Acta Medica Scandinavica* 1955;**5**:371–378.

Little, H. The role of abnormal hemorrheodynamics in the pathogenesis of diabetic retinopathy. *Transactions of the American Ophthalmological Society* 1976;**LXXIV**:573–632.

14. Glasson, P. Traitement de l'hypertension artérielle par plasmaphérèse. *Schweiz Medizinische Wochenschrift/Journal Suisse de Médecine* 1983;**113**:189–191.

15. Walter, U and Distler, A. Abnormal sodium efflux in erythrocyte of patients with essential hypertension. *Hypertension* 1982;**4**:205–210.

Hilton, PJ. Cellular sodium transport in essential hypertension. *New England Journal of Medicine* 1986;**314**:222–229.

Index

The letter *f* following a page number denotes a figure; the letter *t* denotes a table.